Treatment of Non-vitamin K Antagonist Oral Anticoagulants

Masaaki Uno • Kuniaki Ogasawara
Editors

Treatment of Non-vitamin K Antagonist Oral Anticoagulants

For Prevention of Stroke

Springer

Editors
Masaaki Uno
Department of Neurosurgery
Kawasaki Medical School
Kurashiki, Japan

Kuniaki Ogasawara
Department of Neurosurgery
Iwate Medical University
Morioka, Japan

ISBN 978-981-10-1877-0 ISBN 978-981-10-1878-7 (eBook)
DOI 10.1007/978-981-10-1878-7

Library of Congress Control Number: 2016957749

Printed on acid-free paper

This Springer imprint is published by Springer Nature
The registered company is Springer Nature Singapore Pte Ltd.
The registered company address is: 152 Beach Road, #22-06/08 Gateway East, Singapore 189721, Singapore

Preface

I am pleased to present this new textbook, which is targeted at neurologists, neurosurgeons, and doctors who have an interest in stroke. In the pages that follow, information is presented regarding the use of non-vitamin K antagonist oral anticoagulants (NOACs) in stroke patients with a variety of impairments.

In this textbook, the mechanisms, treatment strategies, recurrence rates, outcomes, and complications among stroke patients treated with NOACs are discussed by a variety of different authors. New findings regarding stroke patients in Japan are also included, along with a review of related data from all over the world. It is hoped that readers of this textbook will find not only interesting but also helpful information that can be applied in practice in their own hospitals and clinics. Because the prevalence of nonvalvular atrial fibrillation (NVAF) is increasing around the world, current information and new findings regarding NOACs should be made available to doctors who treat stroke patients with NVAF. I hope that this textbook will serve such a purpose.

Finally, I would like to thank all of the authors for their outstanding contributions, as well as Miss Uchida and Mr. Takayama at Springer Japan for their invaluable assistance in publishing this textbook

Kurashiki, Japan — Masaaki Uno

Preface

I am pleased to present a new textbook entitled *Treatment of NOAC*. Nonvalvular atrial fibrillation represents the most common sustained cardiac arrhythmia and predisposes patients to the development of atrial thrombi, which may embolize to the systemic circulation, particularly the brain. New oral anticoagulant (NOAC) is currently available in the world. Unlike warfarin, these new compounds exhibit a predictable dose response and do not require routine coagulation monitoring, but their anticoagulant effect declines quickly in case of poor compliance, and no coagulation monitoring tests or specific antidotes are currently available. Effectiveness of NOAC has been proved for prophylaxis of stroke in patients with nonvalvular atrial fibrillation using a combined primary outcome of all strokes including intracranial hemorrhage.

Each author in this textbook discusses stroke outcomes, stroke recurrence, and hemorrhagic complications in patients treated with NOACs. In particular, findings regarding intracranial hemorrhagic complications in Japanese people are novel.

I am privileged to have compiled this textbook and am enthusiastic about all that it offers readers. I learned much in the process of editing this book and hope that readers will find this book a uniquely valuable knowledge.

Finally, I would like to thank all of the authors for their outstanding contributions, as well as Miss Uchida and Mr. Takayama at Springer Japan for their invaluable assistance in publishing this textbook.

Morioka, Japan — Kuniaki Ogasawara

Contents

Chapter 1
Secondary Prevention of Stroke with Atrial Fibrillation by New Oral Anticoagulants

K. Kamiyama, T. Osato, and H. Nakamura

Abstract We used the results of secondary prevention analyses for patients with a history of stroke or TIA in the large-scale RE-LY, ROCKET-AF (J-ROCKET-AF), and ARISTOTLE clinical trials to investigate the choice of new oral anticoagulants (NOACs) to prevent recurrent stroke. In light of these results, we concluded that dabigatran 150 mg BID should be the first-choice treatment for comparatively young patients with no apparent renal dysfunction, and apixaban for other patients, and that their efficacy and safety can be broadly guaranteed.

Keywords NVAF (non-valvular atrial fibrillation) • Previous stroke/TIA • Secondary prevention for stroke • Age • Creatinine clearance

1.1 Introduction

According to the results of previous large clinical trials [1–4], new oral anticoagulants (NOACs) showed equivalent or better results to standard anticoagulant treatment with warfarin for the prevention of stroke in patients with non-valvular atrial fibrillation (NVAF) in terms of both efficacy and safety. However, the enrollment criteria and analytical methods used varied somewhat among the studies, and a simple comparison of the results of the use of each drug is therefore inappropriate. There is, however, a need for information on how effective and safe the various NOACs with their different characteristics are in clinical practice.

In this chapter, we focus on the secondary prevention of cardiogenic cerebral embolism in patients with NVAF and discuss the choice of NOAC and treatment policy for preventing recurrent stroke on the basis of the results of subgroup analyses of patients with a history of stroke or TIA in large-scale clinical trials.

K. Kamiyama, M.D. (✉) • T. Osato, M.D. • H. Nakamura, M.D.
Stroke Center, Department of Neurosurgery, Nakamura Memorial Hospital, South-1, West-14, Chuo-ku, Sapporo 060-8570, Japan
e-mail: ikamirin911@med.nmh.or.jp

M. Uno, K. Ogasawara (eds.), *Treatment of Non-vitamin K Antagonist Oral Anticoagulants*, DOI 10.1007/978-981-10-1878-7_1

1.2 Subgroup Analyses of NVAF Patients with a History of Stroke/TIA in Large-Scale Clinical Trials

Once patients with NVAF have experienced a TIA or cerebral infarction, their CHADS2 score increases to ≥2 points, and according to the Japanese guidelines on the management of atrial fibrillation [5], the use of an NOAC is recommended. The results of subgroup analyses of patients with a history of stroke/TIA have been reported from the RE-LY, ROCKET-AF, J-ROCKET-AF, and ARISTOTLE trials [6–9]. The methods of statistical analysis and the presentation used in each trial varied, meaning that a direct comparison cannot be made, but for the sake of simplicity, we quote and analyze the data in the form that they were reported.

1.2.1 A Subgroup Analysis of the RE-LY Trial in Patients with Atrial Fibrillation and Previous Stroke or TIA

The RE-LY trial included 3623 patients with a history of stroke/TIA, accounting for approximately 20 % of the total enrollment. They included 1233 patients treated with dabigatran 110 mg BID, 1233 with dabigatran 150 mg BID, and 1195 with warfarin. The annual incidence of stroke was 2.23 %/year in the dabigatran 110 mg BID arm, 1.91 %/year in the dabigatran 150 mg BID arm, and 2.53 %/year in the warfarin arm, with no significant difference between dabigatran and warfarin. The annual incidence of ischemic or unknown stroke was 2.19 %/year in the 110 mg BID arm, 1.75 %/year in the 150 mg BID arm, and 1.75 %/year in the warfarin arm, with no significant difference between both doses and warfarin, although the rate tended to be somewhat higher in the 110 mg BID arm. For intracranial bleeding, the rates were 0.25 %/year in the 110 mg BID arm, 0.53 %/year in the 150 mg BID arm, and 1.28 %/year in the warfarin arm, with a significant difference between both BID arms and the warfarin arm. For major bleeding, the rates were 2.74 %/year in the 110 mg BID arm, 4.15 %/year in the 150 mg BID arm, and 4.15 %/year in the warfarin arm, with a significant difference for the 110 mg BID arm only [6].

1.2.2 A Subgroup Analysis of the ROCKET-AF Trial in Patients with Atrial Fibrillation and Previous Stroke or TIA

The ROCKET-AF trial included 7468 patients with a history of stroke/TIA, accounting for approximately 52 % of total enrollment. They included 3754 patients treated with rivaroxaban and 3714 with warfarin. The annual incidence of stroke was 2.66 %/year in the rivaroxaban arm and 2.71 %/year in the warfarin arm, with no significant difference between the two arms. The annual incidence of ischemic or unknown stroke was 2.34 %/year in the rivaroxaban arm and 2.27 %/year in the warfarin arm, with no significant difference for this endpoint either. The annual incidence of intracranial bleeding was 0.59 %/year in the rivaroxaban arm and 0.80 %/year in the warfarin arm, slightly lower in the rivaroxaban arm, although this difference was not significant. For major bleeding, the rates were 3.13 %/year in the rivaroxaban arm and 3.22 %/year in the warfarin arm, with no significant difference between the two arms for this parameter either [7].

The J-ROCKET-AF trial of Japanese subjects, who are believed to experience a higher rate of bleeding events as a result of the use of antithrombotics, was a safety validation trial with a smaller dose than the global trial. It included 813 patients with a history of stroke/TIA, accounting for approximately 64 % of the total. Tanahashi et al. carried out an analysis of patients with a history of stroke/TIA [8]. These are valuable data for Japanese patients, but the far lower enrollment compared with other large-scale clinical trials means they should be regarded as reference data. The analysis included 407 patients treated with rivaroxaban and 405 with warfarin. The annual incidence of stroke was 1.47 %/year in the rivaroxaban arm and 3.06 %/year in the warfarin arm, somewhat lower in the rivaroxaban arm, although this difference was not significant. For primary ischemic stroke, the rates were 1.10 %/year in the rivaroxaban arm and 2.48 %/year in the warfarin arm, also lower, but not significantly so. For major bleeding, the rates were 2.40 %/year in the rivaroxaban arm and 3.85 %/year in the warfarin arm, a difference that was also not significant. The endpoints of this particular trial were somewhat different from those of the other large-scale clinical trials, and it has therefore not been included in the forest plot for comparative analysis.

1.2.3 A Subgroup Analysis of the ARISTOTLE Trial Involving Patients with Atrial Fibrillation and Previous Stroke or TIA

The ARISTOTLE trial included 3436 patients with a history of stroke/TIA, accounting for approximately 19 % of total enrollment. They included 1694 patients treated with apixaban and 1742 with warfarin. The annual incidence of stroke was 2.26 %/year in the apixaban arm and 3.17 %/year in the warfarin arm, making this the only reported analysis of secondary stroke prevention to find a significant reduction in the rate of recurrence of stroke in the apixaban arm. The annual incidence of ischemic or unknown stroke was 1.92 %/year in the apixaban arm and 2.23 %/year in the warfarin arm, somewhat lower in the apixaban arm, although this difference was not significant. The annual incidence of intracranial bleeding was 0.55 %/year in the apixaban arm and 1.49 %/year in the warfarin arm, significantly lower in the apixaban arm. Similarly, for major bleeding, the rates were 2.84 %/year in the apixaban arm and 3.91 %/year in the warfarin arm, also significantly lower in the apixaban arm [9].

1.2.4 A Subgroup Analysis of the ENGAGE AF-TIMI 48 Trial Involving Patients with Atrial Fibrillation and Previous Stroke or TIA

The ENGAGE AF-TIMI 48 trial compared edoxaban 30 mg and 60 mg with warfarin [10] and showed that neither arm was inferior to warfarin and that this investigational drug suppressed major bleeding and cardiovascular death. As of March 2016, however, no analysis of secondary prevention for patients with a history of stroke/TIA has yet been published, and edoxaban has therefore been excluded from our analysis in this study.

1.2.5 Hazard Ratios in Each Trial Compared with Warfarin for the Secondary Prevention of Stroke

We extracted data from the results of the subgroup analyses described above and summarized them as a forest plot. To investigate efficacy, we extracted data on stroke and cerebral infarction or stroke of unknown origin and calculated the hazard ratios compared with warfarin (Fig. 1.1). The efficacy of each drug was very similar to that of warfarin, but apixaban was more effective for preventing the recurrence of stroke. We also extracted data on intracranial bleeding and major bleeding in the same way as for our investigation of efficacy and calculated their hazard ratios (Fig. 1.2). This showed that both apixaban and dabigatran 110 mg BID were safer than warfarin.

1.3 Should Efficacy or Safety Be Emphasized in the Secondary Prevention of Stroke?

The decision on which NOAC to use for secondary prevention of stroke in patients with NVAF is an extremely important issue in clinical terms. If the selection criteria are overcomplex, however, this reduces their convenience in clinical use, making them difficult to use as indicators. We therefore considered whether efficacy or safety should be prioritized on the basis of the data from the results of the above subgroup analyses of patients with a history of stroke/TIA, using age and creatinine clearance rate (Ccr) as the XY axes, and we propose simple NOAC selection criteria (Fig. 1.3).

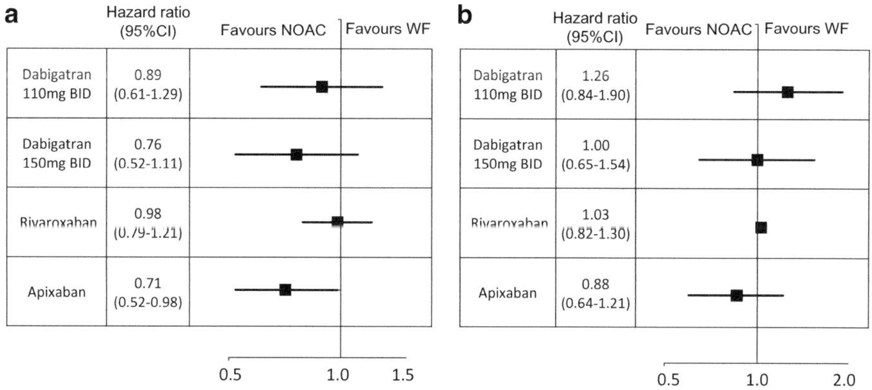

Fig. 1.1 Main efficacy outcomes in patients with previous stroke or TIA among RCTs. (**a**) Stroke. (**b**) Ischemic stroke or unknown type stroke

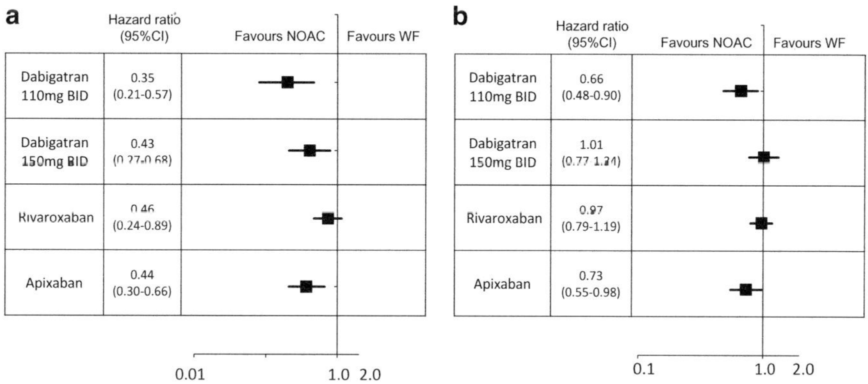

Fig. 1.2 Main safety outcomes in patients with previous stroke or TIA among RCTs. (**a**) Intracranial hemorrhage. (**b**) Major bleeding

This graph has age as its horizontal axis and Ccr as its vertical axis. Ccr values of 30 mL/min and 50 mL/min are important cutoff values for adjusting the dose of each NOAC, and these two lines were therefore drawn as boundary lines. Three of the large-scale clinical trials had also included subgroup analyses by age with 75 years as the boundary, and another boundary line was therefore drawn at age 75 years.

Patients with Ccr >50 mL/min comprise a population with comparatively good renal function and a low rate of hemorrhagic events, and for these patients, efficacy may therefore be prioritized over safety. If Ccr is 30–50 mL/min, hemorrhagic events are a concern, and for this population, safety should be prioritized over efficacy.

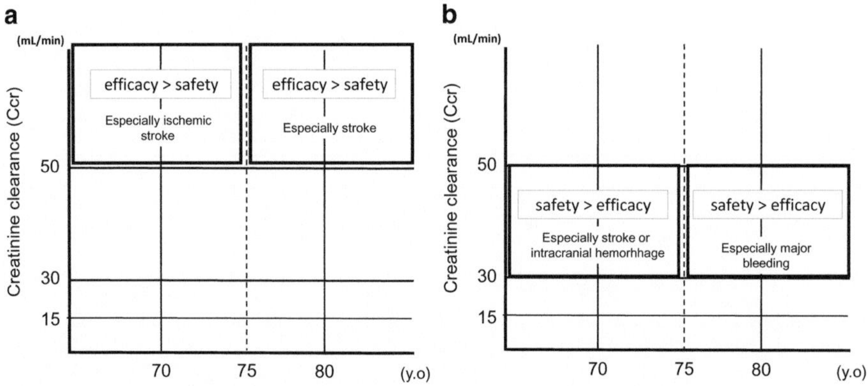

Fig. 1.3 Important factors to consider from age and Ccr in selecting of NOACs. (**a**) Ccr of 51 or more ml/min. (**b**) Ccr of 30–50 ml/min

Patients aged <75 years with Ccr >50 mL/min thus comprise a comparatively young patient population with good renal function. For this group, an NOAC that is more effective in preventing ischemic stroke should therefore be chosen from the subgroup efficacy analyses. Patients aged ≥75 years with Ccr >50 mL/min are elderly, and because hemorrhagic events are a matter of some concern for this group, an NOAC that is more effective in preventing the recurrence of stroke should be chosen from the subgroup efficacy analyses.

For patients aged <75 years with Ccr 30–50 mL/min, efficacy and safety are of around equal importance, and an NOAC that is more effective in preventing the recurrence of stroke but has a lower rate of intracranial bleeding should be chosen. Patients aged ≥75 years with Ccr 30–50 mL/min form an elderly patient population with moderate or worse renal dysfunction, and an NOAC that is more effective in preventing major bleeding should be chosen from the subgroup safety analyses.

1.4 Choice of NOAC for Secondary Stroke Prevention Considered in Light of the Main Analyses and Subgroup Analyses of Large-Scale Clinical Trials (Fig. 1.4)

1.4.1 Patients Aged <75 Years with Ccr >50 mL/min

For patients who fall into this category, efficacy in preventing the recurrence of cerebral infarction is the most important factor to consider. As described above, the secondary prevention analyses show that, at present, no NOAC is more effective than warfarin in preventing the recurrence of cerebral infarction. In the main analysis, however, dabigatran 150 mg BID was more effective in preventing cerebral infarction, and in light of this result, dabigatran 150 mg BID should be chosen as the first-choice medication. In Japan, decreasing the dose of dabigatran from 150 mg

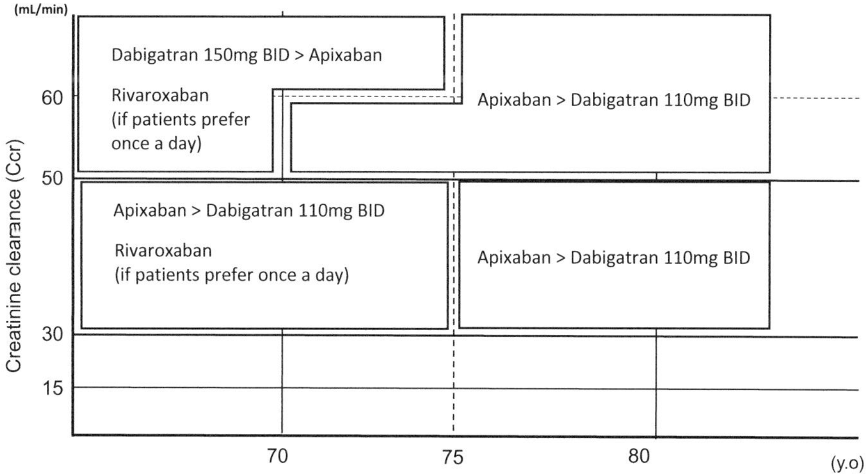

Fig. 1.4 Our clinical guideline in selecting NOACs to patients with previous stroke or TIA

BID must be considered for patients aged ≥70 years. However, patients aged 70–75 years with comparatively good renal function and Ccr well over 50 mL/min (Ccr ≥60 mL/min) re regarded as being at low risk of bleeding, and dabigatran 150 mg BID may therefore be considered. Conversely, a dose of 110 mg BID should perhaps be chosen for patients aged 70–75 years with Ccr only slightly over 50 mL/min. The guidelines created for this category of patients have thus been displayed with *irregularities*. Apixaban should perhaps be considered as a second choice, given that in the secondary prevention analyses, it was the only drug to show greater efficacy than warfarin in preventing the recurrence of stroke. Rivaroxaban should be chosen for patients who prefer to take medication once a day.

1.4.2 Patients Aged ≥75 Years with Ccr >50 mL/min

For patients who fall into this category, efficacy in preventing the recurrence of stroke is the most important aspect of efficacy to consider. In the subgroup analyses of patients with a history of stroke/TIA, apixaban was the only drug that was more effective than warfarin in preventing the recurrence of stroke, and it should therefore be chosen as the first-choice medication. Dabigatran 150 mg BID cannot be used by patients in this category, meaning that the second choice must be dabigatran 110 mg BID. For patients who request a medication that can be taken once a day, the only available choice is rivaroxaban, but the results of an analysis of patients aged ≥75 years in the J-ROCKET-AF trial showed that, in these patients, the rate of severe or clinically significant bleeding was somewhat higher for rivaroxaban than for warfarin. The choice in this case must be made cautiously, and we have not included it in the selection criteria [11].

1.4.3 Patients Aged <75 Years with Ccr 30–50 mL/min

For patients in this category, efficacy in preventing intracranial bleeding is the most important safety-related factor, while preventing the recurrence of stroke is most important in terms of efficacy. Apixaban is more effective than warfarin in preventing intracranial bleeding, and it is also significantly more effective in preventing the recurrence of stroke, making it the first choice for patients in this category. As described in the previous section, dabigatran 150 mg BID cannot be used by patients in this category, meaning that the second choice must be dabigatran 110 mg BID. Rivaroxaban is chosen for patients who request a medication that can be taken once a day.

1.4.4 Patients Aged ≥75 Years with Ccr 30–50 mL/min

For patients in this category, the most important safety-related factor is efficacy in preventing major bleeding. In the subgroup analyses of patients with a history of stroke/TIA, apixaban and dabigatran 110 mg BID were more effective in preventing major bleeding. Between these two, apixaban was also more effective in preventing recurrence of stroke and should perhaps therefore be the first-choice treatment. For many of the patients in this category, however, the dose of apixaban must be adjusted. Almost all data from the ARISTOTLE trial concerned 5 mg BID, and there were few data for 2.5 mg BID. Reliability is therefore considered to be low for a dose of 2.5 mg BID, and dabigatran 110 mg BID should be chosen for patients who require dose adjustment. With respect to rivaroxaban, as described earlier, for patients aged ≥75 years, the rate of severe or clinically significant bleeding was somewhat higher; for patients in this category, it must be administered with caution, and we have not included it in the selection criteria [11].

1.5 Studies of the Choice of NOAC for the Secondary Prevention of Stroke

Several studies have analyzed the question of which of three or four NOACs should be chosen for patients with a history of stroke/TIA in preventing the recurrence of stroke [12–16]. Some of these have recommended rivaroxaban on the grounds that the ROCKET-AF trial enrolled a large number of patients with a history of stroke/TIA. Others, however, have commented that apixaban should be recommended because many patients with a history of stroke/TIA are elderly or suffer from renal dysfunction, and the conclusions vary depending on the viewpoints of the different authors.

1.6 Conclusions

Based on the above results of the subgroup analyses of patients with a history of stroke/TIA, focusing on apixaban in the choice of NOAC for the secondary prevention of stroke enables both efficacy and safety to be broadly guaranteed. However, in clinical practice, this choice should be made cautiously in consideration of the characteristics of the different drugs and the condition of each individual patient.

References

1. Connolly SJ, Ezekowitz MD, Yusuf S, RE-LY Steering Committee and Investigators, et al. Dabigatran versus warfarin in patients with atrial fibrillation. N Engl J Med. 2009;361:1139–51.
2. Patel MR, Mahaffey KW, Garg J, The ROCKET AF Investigators, et al. Rivaroxaban versus warfarin in nonvalvular atrial fibrillation. N Engl J Med. 2011;365:883–91.
3. Hori M, Matsumoto M, Tanahashi N, on behalf of the J-ROCKET AF Study Investigators, et al. Rivaroxaban vs. warfarin in Japanese patients with atrial fibrillation. Circ J. 2012;76:2104–11.
4. Granger CB, Alexander JH, McMurray JJ, ARISTOTLE Committees and Investigators, et al. Apixaban versus warfarin in patients with atrial fibrillation. N Engl J Med. 2011;365:981–92.
5. Joint JCS, Working Group. Guidelines for pharmacotherapy of atrial fibrillation (JCS 2013). Circ J. 2014;78:1997–2021.
6. Diener HC, Connolly SJ, Ezekowitz MD, for the RE LY study group, et al. Dabigatran compared with warfarin in patients with atrial fibrillation and previous transient ischaemic attack or stroke: a subgroup analysis of the RE-LY trial. Lancet Neurol. 2010;9:1157–63.
7. Hankey GJ, Patel MR, Stevens SR, for the ROCKET AF Steering Committee Investigators, et al. Rivaroxaban compared with warfarin in patients with atrial fibrillation and previous stroke or transient ischaemic attack: a subgroup analysis of ROCKET AF. Lancet Neurol. 2012;11:315–22.
8. Tanahashi N, Hori M, Matsumoto M, et al. Rivaroxaban versus warfarin in Japanese patients with nonvalvular atrial fibrillation for the secondary prevention of stroke. J Stroke Cerebrovasc Dis. 2013;22:1317–25.
9. Easton JD, Lopes RD, Bahit MC, for the ARISTOTLE Committees Investigators, et al. Apixaban compared with warfarin in patients with atrial fibrillation and previous stroke or transient ischaemic attack: a subgroup analysis of the ARISTOTLE trial. Lancet Neurol. 2012;11:503–11.
10. Giugliano RP, Ruff CT, Braunwald E, for ENGAGE AF-TIMI 48 Investigators, et al. Edoxaban versus warfarin in patients with atrial fibrillation. N Engl J Med. 2013;28:2093–104.
11. Hori M, Matsumoto M, Tanahashi N, et al. Rivarixaban vs. Warfarin in Japanese patients with non-valvular atrial fibrillation in relation to age: insight from J-ROCKET AF-. Circ J. 2014;78:1349–56.
12. GY L, TB L, Skjøth F, et al. Indirect comparisons of new oral anticoagulant drugs for efficacy and safety when used for stroke prevention in atrial fibrillation. J Am Coll Cardiol. 2012;60:738–46.
13. LH R, TB L, Graungaard T, et al. Primary and secondary prevention with new oral anticoagulant drugs for stroke prevention in atrial fibrillation: indirect comparison analysis. BMJ. 2012;345:e7097.

14. Cairns JA. Which oral anticoagulant for which atrial fibrillation patient: Recent clinical trials and evidence-based choices. Can J Cardiol. 2013;29:1165–72.
15. JI W, J. E. Incorporating edoxaban into the choice of anticoagulants for atrial fibrillation. Thromb Haemost. 2016 Jan;115:257–70.
16. AM S, GY. L. Choosing the right drug to fit the patient when selecting oral anticoagulation for stroke prevention in atrial fibrillation. J Intern Med. 2015;278:1–18.

Chapter 2
Recurrence of Stroke in Patients with AF Using NOACs

Yasushi Ueno

Abstract *Objective*: To evaluate the risk factors of recurrent thromboembolic cerebral infarction in patients with non-valvular atrial fibrillation (NVAF), who were treated with non-vitamin K antagonist oral anticoagulants (NOACs).

Methods: The data of patients is collected from the database of our institute for about 3 years (between 2013 April and 2015 December).

Results: We analyzed 16 patient's data (14 male, 2 female, median age 67.0 years) in whom recurrent thromboembolic cerebral infarction occurred despite receiving NOACs. 14 of 16 patients with recurrent ischemic stroke received reduced dose drug, and in 10 of 14 patient with reduced dose drug, inappropriate dose setting (i.e., out of drug dose criteria of NOACs) has been selected by the physicians or practitioner concerning about the risk for intracranial hemorrhage and patient's age. After we have changed to the appropriate dose, recurrence of thromboembolic cerebral infarction was not observed.

More than 70 % of recurrent cerebral infarction occurred in patients with inappropriate underdose use of NOACs.

Conclusions: This paper demonstrates that patients with inappropriate reduced dose selection of NOACs carry a significant risk of recurrent thromboembolic cerebral infarction despite treated with NOACs anticoagulation, highlighting the need for appropriate drug dose selection for stroke prevention in real-world NVAF patients.

Keywords Recurrent stroke • NOAC • Inappropriate dose setting

---

Y. Ueno (✉)
Department of Neurosurgery and Stroke Center, Shinko Memorial Hospital, 1-4-47 Wakihama-cho, Chuo-ku, Kobe-city, Hyogo 651-0072, Japan
e-mail: yweno@hotmail.co.jp

M. Uno, K. Ogasawara (eds.), *Treatment of Non-vitamin K Antagonist Oral Anticoagulants*, DOI 10.1007/978-981-10-1878-7_2

2.1 Introduction

AF (atrial fibrillation) is a great potential risk factor for cerebral stroke, and AF-associated strokes often lead to severe resulting in disability or death [1–4]. Incidence of AF in the general population ranges from 0.85 to 4.1 per 1000 person-years [5, 6] and increases substantially with age.

Oral anticoagulation with the vitamin K antagonist (VKA) warfarin reduces risk of AF-related thromboembolism and is recommended for a wide number [7] of indications, but how to use this drug is limited by a narrow therapeutic window, drug and food interactions, the need for coagulation monitoring, and the risk of bleeding. According to real-world data, warfarin has been under-used for patients with AF because of high risk of bleeding and intracranial hemorrhage, which lead to the recurrence of any stroke and cerebral infarction [8, 9].

Recently, several non-vitamin K antagonist oral anticoagulants (NOACs) have been developed. Randomized clinical trials (RCTs) comparing NOACs with warfarin demonstrated that NOACs are as safe and effective as warfarin to prevent thromboembolic strokes and systemic embolisms in patients with non-valvular AF (NVAF) [10–14]. Current AF guidelines recommended to use NOACs as first choice [15–17], based on these evidences. Subgroup analysis of the trials indicated that patients with previous stroke or TIA are at high risk of recurrent stroke [1] and of cerebral hemorrhage from anticoagulation therapy [18, 19].

Each NOACs have two types of drug dose, normal dose and reduced dose, and we must select the drug dose based on the patient's age, body weight, and renal function (creatinine clearance: CCr).

Selection criteria for drug dose are different for each NOAC.

The dose of apixaban is 5 mg twice daily or 2.5 mg twice daily for patients with two or more of the following factors: age 80 years or older, body weight 60 kg or less, and serum creatinine 133 μmol/L or greater. ARISTOTLE trial [12] demonstrated that of patients with previous stroke or TIA randomly assigned apixaban, 7 % received the reduced dose (2.5 mg twice daily) and 93 % received the normal dose (5 mg twice daily).

Rivaroxaban is 15 mg daily or 10 mg daily in patients with CCr 30–49 mL/min.

Dabigatran is an oral reversible direct thrombin inhibitor that can be given in fixed daily doses (110 mg or 150 mg twice daily) independent of age or body weight.

However, the analysis reports of real-world thromboembolic stroke recurrence in patients with NVAF using NOACs are rare.

The available RCT shows that in patients on NOACs, the rate of thromboembolic stroke or systemic embolism was 2.07–2.79 per 100 patient-years of follow-up in the NOACs group [10–14, 20].

Analysis of data about stroke recurrence in patients with NOACs can be adequately helpful in the management of stroke survivors who carry high recurrent thromboembolic risk.

The aim of our study is to analyze the real-world data of patients with NVAF who survived a recurrent thromboembolic stroke and in whom anticoagulation therapy with NOACs is treated and to evaluate the mechanisms of recurrence of stroke in NVAF patients using NOACs.

2.2 Materials and Methods

We retrospectively conducted study of patients with NVAF who are treated with anticoagulation therapy with NOACs during 3 years (between 2013 April to 2015 December) after the adoption of NOACs in our hospital.

All patients were treated in the Departments of Neurosurgery and Stroke Center at Shinko Memorial Hospital, Kobe Japan. This study included 16 consecutive patients with NVAF who was afflicted with recurrent thromboembolic cerebral infarction despite using NOACs.

The number of recurrent stroke patients with each NOAC is 2 patients with dabigatran, 10 patients with rivaroxaban, 6 patients with apixaban, and as reference 20 consecutive patients of recurrent cerebral infarction who are treated with warfarin.

To identify patients who were prescribed with NOACs and warfarin, we confirmed each patient's prescription data. We confirmed the diagnosis of NVAF by checking medical records and adherence of drugs by checking the remaining amount of the drugs or interview with patient's family members. Patients with valvular heart disease and thromboembolic infarction of undetermined source were excluded.

The institutional review board of Shinko Memorial Hospital approved this study.

Data on patient age, gender, underlying disease, risk factors, and accompanying medications were obtained from medical records and laboratory data. Creatinine clearance (CCr) was calculated using the Cockcroft–Gault formula [21]. Hypertension was defined as a systolic blood pressure more than 140 mmHg and a diastolic blood pressure more than 90 mmHg. Diabetes mellitus was defined by treatment with hypoglycemic medications or poor glycemic control (defined as a glycohemoglobin A1c more than 6.5 %). Coronary artery disease was defined based on positive stress test results, coronary angiography demonstrating at least 75 % of stenosis, coronary spastic angina documented by an acetylcholine provocation test, a history of prior myocardial infarction, or a history of revascularization procedures. Heart failure was defined according to the American College of Cardiology/American Heart Association criteria [22].

The CHADS2 score (congestive heart failure, hypertension, age more than 75, diabetes, stroke [doubled])and the CHA2DS2-VASc score (congestive heart failure/left ventricular dysfunction, hypertension, age more than 75 [doubled], diabetes, stroke[doubled] – vascular disease – age 65–74, and sex category [female]) were used to measure stroke risk.

HAS-BLED score (hypertension, abnormal renal/liver function [one or two points], stroke, bleeding history or predisposition, labile international normalized ratio, and elderly (>65 years) drugs/alcohol concomitantly [one or two points]) were used to measure hemorrhage risk.

In patients treated with warfarin, we collected prothrombin time-international normalized ratio (PT-INR) data.

Information of patients was obtained from medical records, interview with patient's family members, and the patients' practitioners.

Thromboembolic events included cerebral infarction and transient ischemic attack (TIA). Ischemic cerebral infarction was defined as the sudden onset of a new focal neurological deficit lasting more than 24 h that could not be explained by other causes. TIA was diagnosed when the neurological deficit lasted less than 24 h. Computed tomography or magnetic resonance imaging was performed in all patients.

Statistical analysis summary data were presented either as the mean and standard deviation (SD) and were compared between groups using the Student's t-test and the Mann–Whitney U-test. The cumulative rates of persistence for the prescribed drugs were calculated using the Kaplan–Meier method. Differences in persistence rates were compared using the long rank test. P values less than 0.05 were considered significant.

Data analyses were performed using SPSS statistical software (version11.01, SPSSInc., Chicago, Illinois).

2.3 Results

The clinical database of the usage of each NOACs in our hospital for the 406 patients with NVAF is summarized in Fig. 2.1. Of the 406 patients, 100 (24.7 %) received dabigatran (normal dose 25(25 %); reduced dose 75(75 %)), 130 (32.0 %) received rivaroxaban (normal dose (44.7 %); reduced dose (55.3 %)), and 176 (43.3 %) received apixaban (normal dose (57.4 %); reduced dose (42.6 %)). Of note, in all cases of each NOACs, rates of reduced dose patients were greatly higher compared with that of patients on published RCT data [10–14].

The selection of drug dose was determined by physicians or cardiologist that belongs to our hospital or by practitioner around our hospital, based on the conviction of them.

The reason for the selection of reduced dose NOACs was to avoid drug-induced catastrophic intracranial hemorrhage, especially with elderly patients.

Figure 2.2 demonstrates real-world proportion to select whether normal or reduced dose of rivaroxaban. Fifty-six of 60 (93 %) of patients with CCr ≧50 mL/min and 4 (7 %) with CCr < 50 mL/min received normal dose (15 mg) of rivaroxaban. On the other hand, of note, 39 of 68 (57 %) of patients with CCr ≧50 mL/min and 29 (43 %) with CCr < 50 mL/min received reduced dose (10 mg). These 57 % of patients with CCr ≧50 mL/min, receiving reduced dose of rivaroxaban, should receive normal dose (15 mg). This data demonstrated that inappropriate reduced dose selection of rivaroxaban was 57 % with real-world NVAF patients.

Case: An 87-year-old man was admitted to the emergency room for confused mental status and left-side weakness. He had been treated with reduced dose of

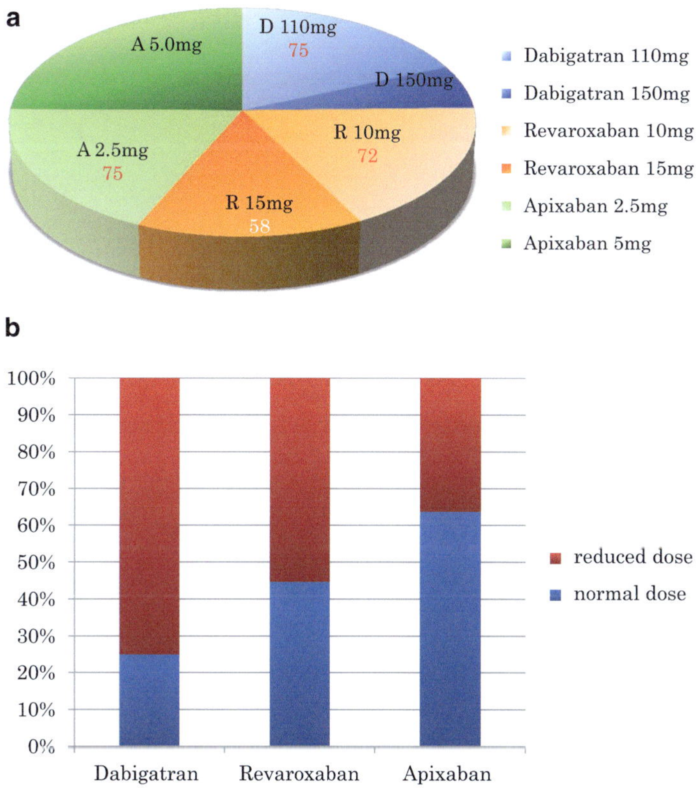

Fig. 2.1 (**a**) The clinical database of the use of each NOAC in our hospital for antithrombotic therapy for the 406 patients with NVAF is summarized in Fig. 2.1. (**b**) Dose selection of 406 patients, dabigatran (normal dose 25(25 %); reduced dose 75(75 %)), rivaroxaban (normal dose (44.7 %); reduced dose (55.3 %)), and apixaban (normal dose (57.4 %); reduced dose (42.6 %)). In all cases of each NOACs, the rate of reduced dose patients was greatly higher compared with that of patients on published RCT data

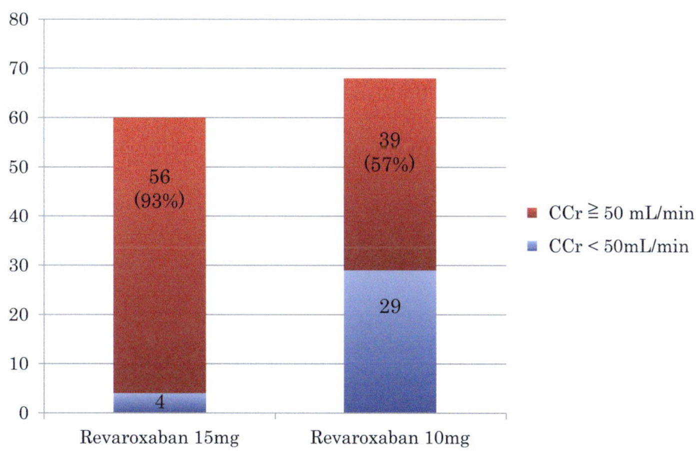

Fig. 2.2 Real-world proportion to select whether normal or reduced dose of rivaroxaban. Thirty-nine of 68 (57 %) of patients with CCr ≧50 mL/min received reduced dose (10 mg). These 57 % of patients with CCr ≧50 mL/min should receive normal dose (15 mg)

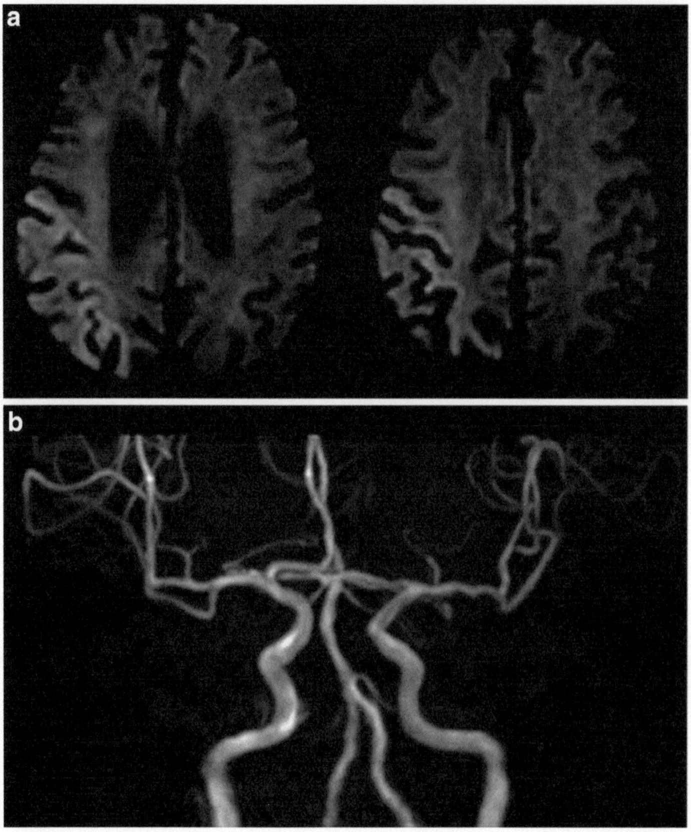

Fig. 2.3 (**a**) Magnetic resonance diffusion weighted imaging revealed acute ischemic infarction in the right middle cerebral artery (MCA) territory. (**b**) Magnetic resonance angiogram imaging revealed no stenosis or occlusion of the right MCA. The patient was diagnosed with TIA due to cardiogenic embolism and recanalization of the occluded MCA in natural course

rivaroxaban (10 mg) for 2 years due to AF and cardiogenic thromboembolic cerebral infarction. He had also been diagnosed and managed for diabetes mellitus. A neurologic examination revealed confused mental status, unresponsiveness to visual threatening, gaze preponderance to the right side, and left-sided hemiparesis. Neurological deficits except slight left motor weakness recovered within several minutes after admission. Magnetic resonance diffusion weighted imaging revealed acute ischemic infarction in the right middle cerebral artery (MCA) territory (Fig. 2.3). The transthoracic echocardiogram findings were consistent with ischemic heart disease with moderate left ventricular systolic dysfunction (left ventricular ejection fraction, 25–30 %), AF with enlargement of both atria, and moderate tricuspid regurgitation. According to coagulation assays on admission, the activated partial thromboplastin time (aPTT) was 38 s (reference, 29.1–41.9 s), and the international normalized ratio (INR) was 1.09 (reference, 0.90–1.10). Magnetic resonance angiogram imaging revealed no stenosis or occlusion of right MCA. He was diagnosed with TIA due to cardiogenic embolism and recanalization of the occluded MCA in natural course.

A baseline assessment revealed that he had a serum creatinine concentration of 0.79 mg/dL and a CCr of 60 mL/min and HAS-BLED score of 2, so he should receive normal dose of rivaroxaban after the onset of previous cerebral infarction.

The decision was made to change from reduced dose of rivaroxaban to normal dose of apixaban because the patient suffered a recurrent ischemic stroke despite receiving rivaroxaban treatment. Apixaban was started at a dosage of 5 mg twice daily, 2 days after the cessation of rivaroxaban. The patient improved and completely recovered without any neurological deficit, and no recurrent of ischemic stroke was observed after 6 months of apixaban usage.

Figure 2.4 demonstrated real-world proportion to select whether normal or reduced dose of each NOAC for the NVAF patients with recurrent cerebral infarction despite receiving NOACs.

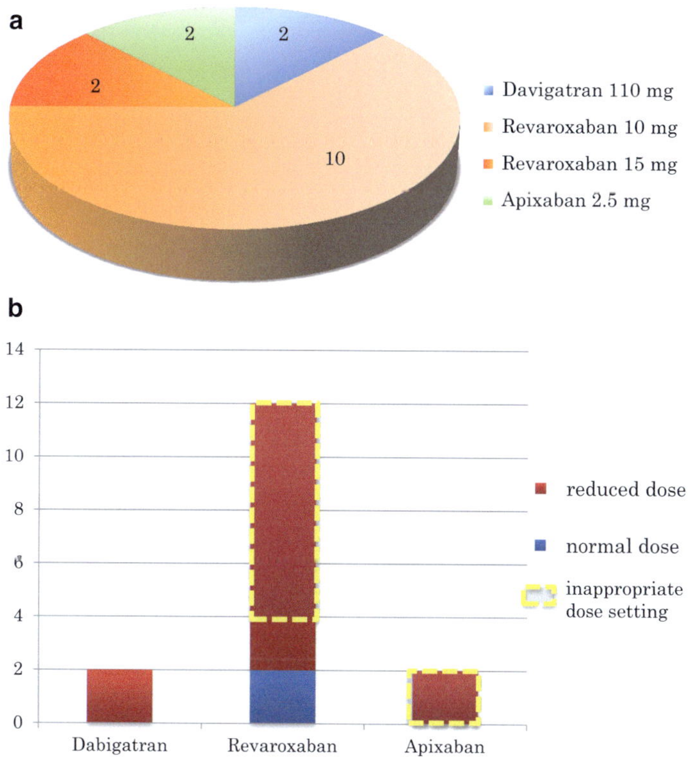

Fig. 2.4 (**a**) Real-world proportion to select whether normal or reduced dose of each NOACs for the NVAF patients with recurrent cerebral infarctions. (**b**) Eight of ten patients with reduced dose should receive normal dose (15 mg daily) based on the drug dose criteria of rivaroxaban. Similarly, all of two patients with recurrent stroke despite using apixaban received reduced dose (2.5 mg twice daily) drug and should receive normal dose (5 mg twice daily) based on the drug dose criteria of apixaban

Ten of 12 NVAF patients with recurrent stroke despite using rivaroxaban received reduced dose (10 mg daily) drug, and 8 of 10 patients with reduced dose should receive normal dose (15 mg daily) based on the drug dose criteria of rivaroxaban.

Similarly, all of two patients with recurrent stroke despite using apixaban received reduced dose (2.5 mg twice daily) drug and should receive normal dose (5 mg twice daily) based on the drug dose criteria of apixaban.

Two patients with recurrent stroke despite using dabigatran received reduced dose (110 mg) drug, but dabigatran can be given in fixed daily doses (110 mg or 150 mg twice daily) independent of age or body weight.

To summarize the above data, 14 of 16 patients with recurrent ischemic stroke, despite of using NOACs, received reduced dose drug, and in 10 of 14 patient with reduced dose drug, inappropriate dose setting (i.e., out of drug dose criterion of NOACs) has been selected by the physicians or practitioner.

After we have changed to the appropriate dose, the recurrence of thromboembolic cerebral infarction was not observed.

More than 70 % of recurrent cerebral infarction occurred in patients with inappropriate underdose use of NOACs.

2.4 Discussion

2.4.1 Warfarin Versus NOACs

The main aim of anticoagulant therapy in a patient of AF is to avoid consequences of arterial thrombus formation, including peripheral embolism, especially cerebral infarction.

Considering the growing number of AF patients and the fact that AF occurs in 15 % of the whole stroke population, the importance of both effective and safe antithrombotic treatment should be emphasized [23–25]. According to previously performed RCTs and guidelines, the application of oral anticoagulants is recommended for stroke prevention in AF patients [8–14].

For many years, VKA was used in that patient group, resulting in a significant stroke rate reduction exceeding the efficacy of antiplatelet treatment [8, 9].

Significant problems related to anticoagulant therapy with VKA are high rate of intracranial hemorrhage, relatively narrow therapeutic window and poor adherence, drug and food interactions, and the need for coagulation monitoring [26].

So, despite the high rate of stroke in patients with AF, an even smaller proportion of patients are properly treated with anticoagulants, which lead to the recurrence of any stroke and cerebral infarction [8, 9].

The introduction of NOACs creates a potential opportunity to bridge the gap between the need of anticoagulant treatment and practice application of this kind of therapy.

That could result not only in high-treatment efficacy but also in obtaining higher rates of successful anticoagulant treatment in AF patients with proper anticoagulant protection.

According to the RCTs inducted, high efficacy and safety of NOACs was documented in patients with NVAF [10–14]. At least the non-inferiority efficacy and safety of NOACs in the prevention of stroke and systemic embolism was documented in studies, as compared with VKA studies [10–14].

An encouraging safety profile, especially in the aspect of intracranial hemorrhage, was simultaneously confirmed. The promising results of randomized trials were also confirmed in meta-analyses [10–14]. Recently published meta-analyses related to NOACs in NVAF demonstrated that the benefit of NOAC use was greater than that of warfarin in terms of stroke reduction and systemic embolism.

According to the results from the Danish Registry [27], the mortality among patients using NOACs was lower than among those treated with VKA.

2.4.2 Frequency of Anticoagulants Use

According to the randomized clinical trials of effects of antithrombotic therapy in patients with NVAF [5], warfarin use has increased gradually. Previously warfarin was used for 8–17 % of patients with AF [28] but had increased to 51.7 % of NVAF patients in the present study. Approximately 50 % of NVAF patients with high risk of embolism received anticoagulation with warfarin; that is, anticoagulant use is still insufficient among patients with NVAF treated by cardiologists and practitioners. The intensities of warfarin therapy in the previous reviews were slightly lower than those recommended by the guideline [29]. The under-use of anticoagulant warfarin might be based on data from prospective, secondary prevention trials [30].

In many NVAF patients, the antithrombotic therapy did not follow the guideline [29]. Warfarin, rather than other antiplatelet drugs like aspirin, was used more frequently to patients aged 75 years old or younger. Only one fifth of patients aged over 75 years were given warfarin. In previous studies, warfarin use was less frequent for older patients [31]; that was because of high risk of major bleeding and other complications in the elderly patients; however, warfarin can be used safely and efficiently among older patients (over 90 years old) without any risk factors for intracranial bleeding.

2.4.3 Under-Use of Warfarin and NOACs

First, based on clinical trials, an INR of 2–3 is recommended to prevent thromboembolic events in patients with NVAF [29], but for Japanese patients, an INR of 1.6–2.6 is considered appropriate, based on prospective, secondary prevention trials [30]. This narrow therapeutic window might lead to the inconvenience of INR monitoring and poor patient adherence. However, several studies about the relationship between INR score and stroke or bleeding risk have shown that an INR of below 2.0 is associated with a greater increase in the risk of stroke than the increase in the risk of bleeding associated with an INR of more than 3.0 [32, 33].

Second, previous studies indicate that approximately 50–60 % of NVAF patients do not have contraindications to anticoagulation with warfarin, and the risk of bleeding seems the most frequent cause of hesitation in using warfarin [34].

Surprisingly, there were approximately 30 % of NVAF patients with risk factors for embolism, who did not have any apparent reasons for the nonuse or under-use of warfarin including paroxysmal AF in the study by Bradley et al. [35].

Patients with atrial fibrillation and prior stroke or transient ischemic attack were found to be undertreated with NOAC anticoagulation therapy in this study, similar to the cases of VKA warfarin. All guidelines recommend that AF patients at high risk for stroke should receive anticoagulation therapy with warfarin; however, despite the effective prophylaxis of warfarin, patients with AF at high risk for stroke are often undertreated.

The Euro-Heart Survey, the study of stroke prevention in AF in 35 European countries, concluded that real-world antithromboembolic therapy in AF patients was not well tailored to the patient's stroke risk profile [26]; additionally, a US population-based study reported that 41 % of AF patients at high risk for stroke did not receive warfarin [36].

The under-use of oral anticoagulation therapy in the AF patients may have many reasons [37–39]. These include low levels of therapy initiation, the narrow therapeutic window (INR 2–3 in NVAF) leading to the inconvenience of INR monitoring, and patient adherence, and especially fear of drug-induced renal dysfunction and catastrophic intracranial hemorrhage might contribute to the NOAC underutilization for AF as well as warfarin.

In this respect, the results of postregistration observational studies related to real-world efficacy and safety are also important. We analyzed the results of 18 NVAF patients with recurrent cerebral infarction treated by the means of NOACs in a real-world clinical setting. Our study indicated that in 16 of 18 patients, the dose of drugs was reduced, and in 14 of 16 patients with reduced dose drugs, inappropriate dose setting has been selected by the physicians or practitioner concerning about the risk for bleeding or drug-induced renal dysfunction based on the conviction of them.

Actually we observed major bleeding in the patients with NOACs; however, the definition of major bleeding differed from each studies and the validity of the comparison is limited. Predictors for bleeding in patients with anticoagulants include many clinical factors, such as history of myocardial infarction, ischemic heart disease, uncontrolled hypertension, previous cerebrovascular disease, anemia or a history of systemic bleeding, and, what is most important, concomitant use of anticoagulant such as antiplatelet agents like aspirin [40].

Some studies show no increase in bleeding with increasing age [41]; the other analysis clearly demonstrated that increasing age raises the risk of intracranial bleeding [42]. In addition, the increased risk of bleeding with oral anticoagulants was far smaller than the beneficial reduction in risk of stroke [42].

Importantly, in AF patients, some risk factors like diabetes mellitus, controlled hypertension, and gender for anticoagulation-related bleeding are also indications for the use of anticoagulants.

Our study indicated that the inappropriate under-use of NOACs is greatly related to high risk of recurrent cerebral infarction in AF patients in real-world clinical practice and reflects the need for improvements in setting appropriate drug dose of NOACs for high-risk patients with AF.

2.4.4 Limitations

First, in these analyses, patient's economical context, patients' refusal, and their life expectancy were not included as reasons for nonuse or under-use of NOACs. Second, the incidence of intracranial hemorrhage is greatly higher in Japanese subjects than in Caucasian subject [43], which could lead, at least in part, to the under-use of NOACs. Third, the present data were collected from only our hospital and might not represent nationwide trends of NOAC use in Japan. Finally, patients being treated with non-anticoagulant therapies (antiplatelets, such as aspirin) might mitigate the strength of a general claim of "under-use treatment."

2.5 Conclusions

Real-world clinical benefit of NOACs resulted in the high efficacy and acceptable safety in the treatment of patient with NVAF, if we use NOACs with proper dosage, but under-use of NOACs leads to high rate of stroke recurrence. This paper demonstrates the under-use of NOACs for real-world NVAF patients with an elevated risk of recurrent stroke, highlighting the need for appropriate drug dose selection for stroke prevention in NVAF patients.

References

1. Wolf PA, Abbott RD, Kannel WB. Atrial fibrillation as an independent risk factor for stroke: the Framingham Heart Study. Stroke 1991; 22:983–988.
2. Atrial Fibrillation Investigators. Risk factors for stroke and efficacy of antithrombotic therapy in atrial fibrillation. Analysis of pooled data from five randomized controlled trials. Arch Intern Med 1994;154:1449–1457.
3. Hughes M, Lip GY. Stroke and thromboembolism in atrial fibrillation: a systematic review of stroke risk factors, risk stratification schema and cost effectiveness data. Thromb Haemost 2008;99:295–304.
4. Stroke in Atrial Fibrillation Working Group. Independent predictors of stroke in patients with atrial fibrillation: a systematic review. Neurology 2007;69:546–554.
5. Murphy NF, Simpson CR, Jhund PS, et al. A national survey of the prevalence, incidence, primary care burden and treatment of atrial fibrillation in Scotland. Heart. 2007;93:606–12.

6. Miyasaka Y, Barnes ME, Gersh BJ, et al. Secular trends in incidence of atrial fibrillation in Olmsted County, Minnesota, 1980 to 2000, and implications on the projections for future prevalence. Circulation. 2006;114:119–25.
7. Hart RG, Pearce LA, Aguilar MI. Meta-analysis: antithrombotic therapy to prevent stroke in patients who have nonvalvular atrial fibrillation. Ann Intern Med 2007;146:857–867.
8. Ogilvie IM, Newton N, Welner SA, et al. Underuse of oral anticoagulants in atrial fibrillation: a systemic review. Am J Med 2010;123:638–645.
9. Inoue H, Nozawa T, Okumura K, et al. Attitudes of Japanese cardiologists toward anticoagulation for nonvalvular atrial fibrillation and reasons for its underuse. Circ J. 2004;68:417–21.
10. Connolly SJ, Ezekowitz MD, Yusuf S, et al. Dabigatran versus warfarinin patients with atrial fibrillation. N Engl J Med. 2009;361:1139–51.
11. Patel MR, Mahaffey KW, Garg J, et al. Rivaroxaban versus warfarin in nonvalvular atrial fibrillation. N Engl J Med. 2011;365:883–91.
12. Granger CB, Alexander JH, McMurray JJ, et al. Apixaban versus warfarin in patients withatrial fibrillation. N Engl J Med. 2011;365:981–92.
13. Giugliano RP, Ruff CT, Braunwald E, et al. Once-daily edoxaban versus warfarin in patients with atrial fibrillation. N Engl J Med. 2013;369:2093–104.
14. Ruff CT, Giugliano RP, Braunwald E, et al. Comparison of the efficacy and safety of new oral anticoagulants with warfarin in patients with atrial fibrillation: a meta-analysis of randomized trials. Lancet. 2014;383:955–62.
15. Skanes AC, Healey JS, JA C, et al. Focused 2012 update of the Canadian Cardiovascular Society atrial fibrillation guidelines: recommendations for stroke prevention and rate/ rhythm control. Can J Cardiol. 2012;28:125–36.
16. Camm AJ, Lip GY, DeCaterina R, et al. 2012 Focused update of theESC Guidelines for the management of atrial fibrillation: an update of the2010ESC Guidelines for the management of atrial fibrillation. Developed with the special contribution of the European Heart Rhythm Association. Eur Heart J. 2012;33:2719–47.
17. JCS Joint Working Group. Guidelines for pharmaco therapy of atrial fibrillation (JCS 2013)-digest version. Circ J. 2014;78:1997–2021.
18. EAFT (European Atrial Fibrillation Trial) Study Group. Secondary prevention in non-rheumatic atrial fibrillation after transient ischaemic attack or minor stroke. Lancet. 1993;342:1255–62.
19. Gorter JW. Major bleeding during anticoagulation after cerebral ischemi: patterns and risk factors. Stroke Prevention In Reversible Ischemia Trial (SPIRIT). European Atrial Fibrillation Trial (EAFT) study groups. Neurology. 1999;53:1319–27.
20. Lopes RD, Alexander JH, Al-Khatib SM, et al. Apixaban for reduction in stroke and other thromboembolic events in atrial fi brillation (ARISTOTLE) trial: design and rationale. Am Heart J. 2010;159:331–9.
21. Cockcroft DW, Gault MH. Prediction of creatinine clearance from serum creatinine. Nephron. 1976;16:31–41.
22. Hunt SA, Abraham WT, Chin MH, et al. Focused update in corporated into the ACC/AHA 2005 guidelines for the diagnosis and management of heart failure in adults: A report of the American College of Cardiology Foundation/American Heart Association Task Force on Practice Guide lines. Circulation. 2009;119:e391–479.
23. Fang MC, Go AS, Chang Y, et al. Warfarin discontinuation after starting warfarin for atrial fibrillation. Circ Cardiovasc Qual Outcomes. 2010;3:624–31.
24. Sorensen SV, Dewilde S, Singer DE, et al. Cost-effectiveness of warfarin: trial versus "real-world" stroke prevention in atrial fibrillation. Am Heart J. 2009;157:1064–73.
25. Gallego P, Roldan V, Marin F, et al. Cessation of oral anticoagulation in relation to mortality and the risk of thrombotic events in patients with atrial fibrillation. Thromb Haemost. 2013;110:1189–98.
26. Nieuwlaat R, Capucci A, Lip GY, et al. Antithrombotic treatment in real-life atrial fibrillation patients: a report from the Euro Heart Survey on Atrial Fibrillation. Eur Heart J. 2006;27:3018–26.

27. Banerjee A, Lane DA, Torp-Pedersen C, Lip GY. Net clinical benefiet of new oral anlticoagulants (dabigadran, rivaroxaban, apixaban) versus no treatment in a 'real world' AF population: a modelling analysis based on a nationwide cohort study. Thromb Hacmost. 2012;107:584–9.
28. Research Group for Antiarrhythmic Drug Therapy. Survey of atrial fibrillation and thromboembolism in the elderly: A multicenter coop- erative study. J Cardiol. 1999;33:27–35.
29. Cairns JA. Atrial fibrillation: Antithrombotic therapy. In: Yusuf S, Cairns JA, Camm AJ, Fallen EL, Gersh BJ, editors. Evidence-based cardiology. London: BMJ Books; 1998. p. 544–52.
30. Yasaka M, Minematsu K, Yamaguchi T. Optimal intensity of inter- national normalized ratio in warfarin therapy for secondary prevention of stroke in patients with non-valvular atrial fibrillation. Intern Med. 2001;40:1183–8.
31. McCrory DC, Matchar DB, Samsa G, Sanders LL, Pritchett ELC. Physician attitudes about anticoagulation for nonvalvular atrial fibril- lation in the elderly. Arch Intern Med. 1995;155:277–81.
32. Hylek EM, Go AS, Chang Y, et al. Effect of intensity of oral antico- agulation on stroke severity and mortality in atrial fibrillation. N Engl J Med. 2003;349:1019–26.
33. Hylek EM, Singer DE. Risk factors for intracranial hemorrhage in outpatients taking warfarin. Ann Intern Med. 1994;120:897–902.
34. Smith NL, Psaty BM, Furberg CD, White R, Lima JA, Newman AB, et al. Temporal trends in the use of anticoagulants among older adults with atrial fibrillation. Arch Intern Med. 1999;159:1574–8.
35. Bradley BC, Perdue KS, Tisdel KA, Gilligan DM. Frequency of anticoagulation for atrial fibrillation and reasons for its non-use at a veterans affairs medical center. Am J Cardiol. 2000;85:568–72.
36. Glazer NL, Dublin S, Smith NL, et al. Newly detected atrial fibrillation and compliance with antithrombotic guidelines. Arch Intern Med. 2007;167:246–52.
37. Reynolds MR, Shah J, Essebag V, et al. Patterns and predictors of warfarin use in patients with new-onset atrial fibrillation from the FRACTAL Registry. Am J Cardiol. 2006;97:538–43.
38. Gattellari M, Worthington J, Zwar N, et al. Barriers to the use of anticoagulation for nonvalvular atrial fibrillation: a representative survey of Australian family physicians. Stroke. 2008; 39: 227-230.
39. Anderson N, Fuller R, Dudley N. 'Rules of thumb' or reflective practice? Understanding senior physicians' decision-making about antithrombotic usage in atrial fibrillation. QJM. 2007;100:263–9.
40. Hughes M, Lip GY. Risk factors for anticoagulation-related bleeding complications in patients with atrial fibrillation: A systematic review. QJM. 2007;100:599–607.
41. McNamara RL, Tamariz LJ, Segal JB, et al. Management of atrial fibrillation: Review of the evidence for the role of pharmacologic therapy, electrical cardioversion, and echocardiography. Ann Intern Med. 2003;139:1018–33.
42. van Walraven C, Hart RG, Connolly S, et al. Effect of age on stroke prevention therapy in patients with atrial fibrillation. The Atrial Fibrillation Investigators. Stroke. 2009;40:1410–6.
43. Tanaka H, Hayashi M, Date C, Imai K, Asada M, Shoji H, et al. Epidemiologic studies of stroke in Shibata, a Japanese provincial city: Preliminary report on risk factors for cerebral infarction. Stroke. 1985;16:773–80.

Chapter 3
Intracranial Bleeding

Masahiro Yasaka

Abstract The non-vitamin K antagonist oral anticoagulants (NOACs), dabigatran, rivaroxaban, apixaban, and edoxaban, are associated with a much lower incidence of intracranial hemorrhage than warfarin. This may be due to the fact that NOACs do not affect plasma concentrations of factor VII or the complexes of tissue factor and factor VIIa that are essential for the first reaction in the coagulation cascade, whereas warfarin suppresses factor VII production even within the therapeutic range of prothrombin time-international normalized ratios (PT-INRs). Another explanation may be that there are fewer coagulation inhibition points in the coagulation cascade with NOAC treatment than with warfarin treatment, and NOACs have a trough phase, while warfarin does not. There may be differences in the sites preventing intracranial hemorrhage between thrombin inhibitors and Xa inhibitors. Data have indicated that thrombin inhibitors and Xa inhibitors more strongly suppress brain hemorrhage and subdural hematoma, respectively, than warfarin. Analysis of the results obtained for East Asians in Phase III trials showed that, though the warfarin dose was maintained at a lower level for East Asians, the incidence of intracranial hemorrhage was higher among East Asians than non-East Asians. However, when an NOAC is used instead of warfarin, there is greater reduction of the incidence of intracranial hemorrhage in East Asians than in non-East Asians. Nonsurgical measures for intracranial hemorrhage during NOAC treatment are general measures, including systolic blood pressure control to less than 140 mmHg, charcoal administration, and application of hemodialysis to remove dabigatran, and specific measures, such as coagulation factor therapy including four-factor prothrombin complex concentrate, recombinant activated factor VII, and several antidotes including idarucizumab, andexanet alfa, and ciraparantag (arapazine).

Keywords Non-vitamin K antagonist oral anticoagulants (NOACs) • Intracranial hemorrhage • Antidote • East Asia • Coagulation cascade

---

M. Yasaka, M.D., Ph.D. (✉)
Department of Cerebrovascular Medicine and Neurology, National Hospital Organization, Kyushu Medical Center, 1-8-1 Jigyohama, Chuo-ku, Fukuoka 810-8563, Japan
e-mail: yasaka@kyumed.jp

M. Uno, K. Ogasawara (eds.), *Treatment of Non-vitamin K Antagonist Oral Anticoagulants*, DOI 10.1007/978-981-10-1878-7_3

3.1 Introduction

Intracranial bleeding (ICH) consists of hemorrhagic stroke, including brain hemorrhage and subarachnoid hemorrhage, and trauma-related hemorrhage, such as chronic subdural hematoma and acute epidural hematoma. ICH is one of the major causes of death and disability. Antithrombotic agents are strongly related to the pathology and prognosis of ICH. However, since non-vitamin K antagonist oral anticoagulants (NOACs) appeared (Table 3.1), the features of ICH have been shown to differ markedly between warfarin and NOAC treatment, and the superiority of NOACs over warfarin has been clearly demonstrated. This article summarizes the features of ICH with antithrombotic agents, warfarin or NOACs, in East Asians and Non-East Asians, prevention of brain hemorrhage, and nonsurgical measures at the time of occurrence of ICH during NOAC treatment.

3.2 Intracranial Bleeding During Antithrombotic Therapy in the Warfarin Era

Prior antithrombotic therapy with antiplatelet agents, warfarin, or both was found to be associated with the location of cerebellar hemorrhage, lobar hemorrhage, and thalamic hemorrhage, large hematoma, hematoma enlargement, and poor prognosis with early death in Japanese patients with intracranial hemorrhage (Fig. 3.1) [1–4].

Itabashi et al. investigated the relationship between antithrombotic therapy and the anatomical location of acute brain hemorrhage in 484 consecutive patients with an acute brain hemorrhage and found that bleeding in the thalamus (44.8 % vs. 30.7%), cerebellum (7.8 %, vs. 2.7 %), and brain lobes (18.1 % vs. 11.4 %) was more frequently seen in 116 patients with prior antithrombotic therapy than in the other 368 patients without ($p < 0.0001$) [2].

Table 3.1 Characteristics of thrombin inhibitors and Xa inhibitors

	Dabigatran	Rivaroxaban	Apixaban	Edoxaban
Target factor	Thrombin	Xa	Xa	Xa
Half-life time (h)	12–14	9–13	8–15	6–11
T max (h)	0.5–2	2–4	1–4	1–1.5
Bioavailability	6.5 %(humans)	67–86 % (animal)	49 % (human)	60 % (animals)
Protein binding	35 %	92–95 %	87 %	40–50 %
Metabolism	Glucuronidation	CYP3A4/2J2	CYP3A4	CYP3A
Renal excretion	80 %	33 %	25 %	35–39 %
Prodrug	Yes	No	No	No
Company	Boehringer	Bayer	Bristol-Myer	Daiichi Sankyo
	Ingelheim		Squibb/Pfizer	

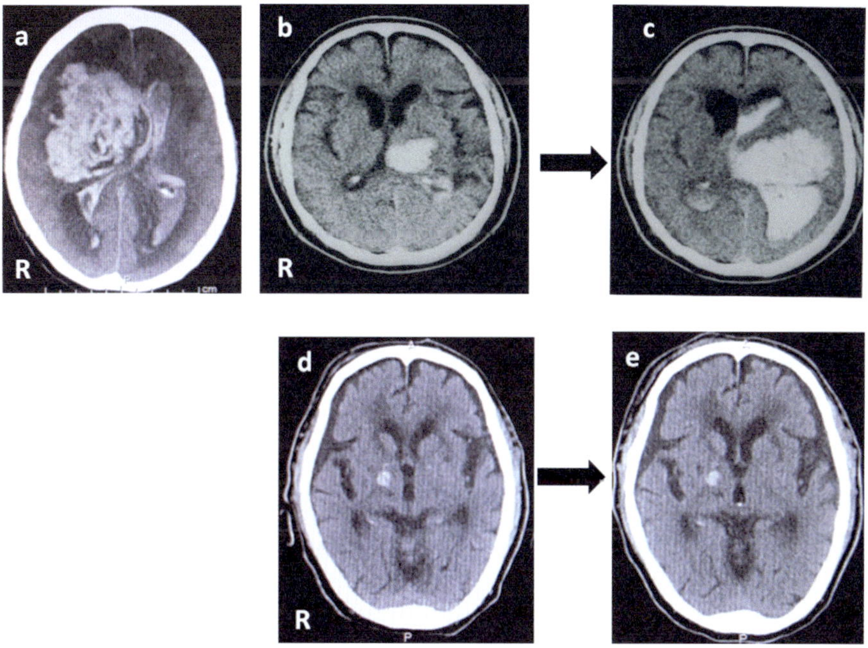

Fig. 3.1 ICH during anticoagulant therapy with warfarin or NOAC
Brain CT images of an acute intracerebral hemorrhage during warfarin (*upper*) or NOAC (*lower*) treatment. (**a**): Large hematoma at the *right* putamen. (**b**) and (**c**): Enlargement of the *left* thalamic hemorrhage. (**d**) and (**e**): Small hematoma at the *right* thalamus has not expanded

Toyoda et al. examined whether the use of oral antithrombotic agents before the onset of intracerebral hemorrhage affected hematoma features and early patient outcomes in 1006 patients with acute intracerebral hemorrhage, including 180 with prior antiplatelet therapy, 67 with prior warfarin therapy, and 21 with both, and they demonstrated that taking each kind of antithrombotic agent was independently related to hematoma enlargement within the initial 24 hours and mortality at 3 weeks after the onset of intracerebral hemorrhage [3].

Kuwashiro et al. compared hematoma size between 41 patients having acute brain hemorrhage with and 323 without prior warfarin therapy, and they found that both hematoma volume on admission and final volume were significantly larger, and both hematoma enlargement and early death within 30 days were more frequently seen with than without prior warfarin therapy [4].

3.3 NOACs vs. Warfarin

3.3.1 Incidence and Features of ICH

Phase III trials of NOACs have demonstrated a much lower incidence of intracranial hemorrhage in patients treated with NOACs than in those treated with warfarin (Fig. 3.2) [5–10]. Graham et al. investigated the comparative safety of dabigatran and warfarin in a general practice setting using Medicare data in the United States and found that dabigatran was associated with a reduced risk of intracranial hemorrhage [11]. Komori et al. retrospectively reviewed the clinical data and treatment summaries of nine intracranial bleeds (two intracerebral bleeds) that developed during dabigatran treatment in eight patients with non-valvular atrial fibrillation; they found that hematomas arising due to acute intracranial bleeding during dabigatran treatment seemed to remain small to moderate, tended not to expand much, and were manageable [12].

Hagii et al. studied the characteristics of ICH during rivaroxaban treatment by comparison with ICH during warfarin treatment [13]. They compared ICH in five patients treated with rivaroxaban and in 56 patients treated with warfarin, and they found that patients with rivaroxaban-associated ICH developed relatively small hematomas, showed no expansion of the hematoma, and had favorable functional outcomes compared with those with warfarin-associated ICH.

Hylek et al. investigated the ARISTOTLE data for mortality in patients with major hemorrhage and found that, compared with warfarin, apixaban was associated with fewer intracranial hemorrhages, less severe adverse consequences

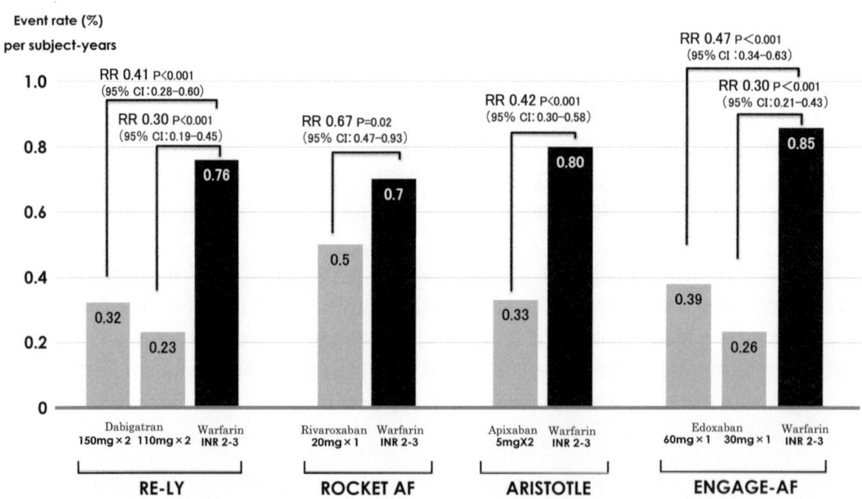

Fig. 3.2 Incidence of intracranial hemorrhage in Phase III trials of NOACs
The incidence of hemorrhagic stroke is much lower with each NOAC treatment than with warfarin, quoted from Refs. [5–8]

following extracranial hemorrhages, and a 50 % reduction in fatal consequences at 30 days in cases of major hemorrhage [14]. One of the reasons for the favorable outcomes in patients with major hemorrhage during apixaban treatment may be that hematomas occurring during apixaban treatment tend to show limited expansion.

3.3.2 Hemostatic Background

One of the reasons why the incidence of ICH was much lower in the NOAC treatment group than in the warfarin treatment group may be attributable to the characteristics of NOACs, which have a short half-life of around half a day and do not affect plasma concentrations of factor VII or the complexes of tissue factor and factor VIIa that are essential for the first reaction in the coagulation cascade, whereas warfarin suppresses factor VII production even within the therapeutic range of prothrombin time-international normalized ratios (PT-INRs), resulting in a higher rate of ICH (Fig. 3.3) [15–17]. The next reason is the fact that there are fewer coagulation inhibition points in the coagulation cascade with NOAC treatment than with warfarin treatment. Warfarin suppresses the production of four coagulation factors, namely, factors II, VII, IX, and X. On the other hand, both thrombin inhibitors and Xa inhibitors have inhibitory actions on only one coagulation factor. This perhaps provides fewer chances of hemorrhage than with warfarin. Another reason could be

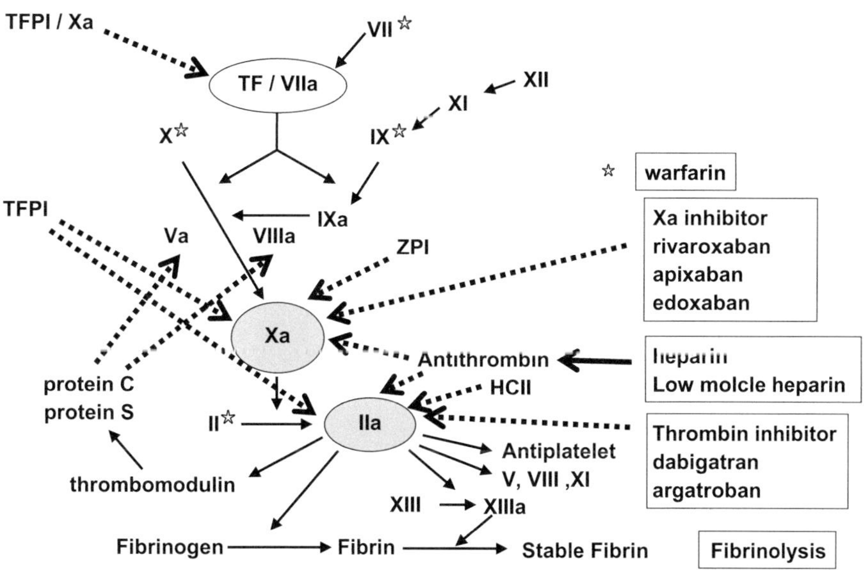

Fig. 3.3 The coagulation cascade and the sites of action of anticoagulants
The solid lines indicate promoting action and the dotted lines inhibitory action
TF tissue factor, *TFPI* tissue factor pathway inhibitor, *ZPI* protein Z induced protease inhibitor, *HCII* heparin cofactor II

the difference in the safe dose range, which is wide for NOACs and narrow for warfarin [18]. Changes in the blood concentrations of the drug may also have some effect. Warfarin does not show major diurnal changes in its effect, but NOACs, which have a half-life of about 12 h, show peak and trough concentrations. During the troughs, NOACs do not have a strong suppressive effect on biological hemostasis, which is probably related to the lower incidence of hemorrhage. The mechanism of the lower incidence of intracranial hemorrhage perhaps explains why hematomas do not grow much in patients receiving NOAC treatment (Fig. 3.1).

3.3.3 *Thrombin vs. Xa Inhibitors*

It is obvious that both thrombin and Xa inhibitors have a much lower incidence of intracranial hemorrhage than warfarin [1–4]. However, there may be differences in the site of preventing intracranial hemorrhage between the two types of NOACs. Comparative data on hemorrhagic stroke, including mainly brain hemorrhage and a few cases of subarachnoid hemorrhage, between NOAC and warfarin showed an outstandingly low incidence of hemorrhagic stroke with dabigatran compared to warfarin [1–4, 19] (Fig. 3.4).

Saji et al. conducted a multicenter, retrospective, cohort study in Japan to elucidate the pathophysiology of intracranial hemorrhage associated with NOACs and found that the proportion of cerebral hemorrhage in ICH was lower with dabigatran than

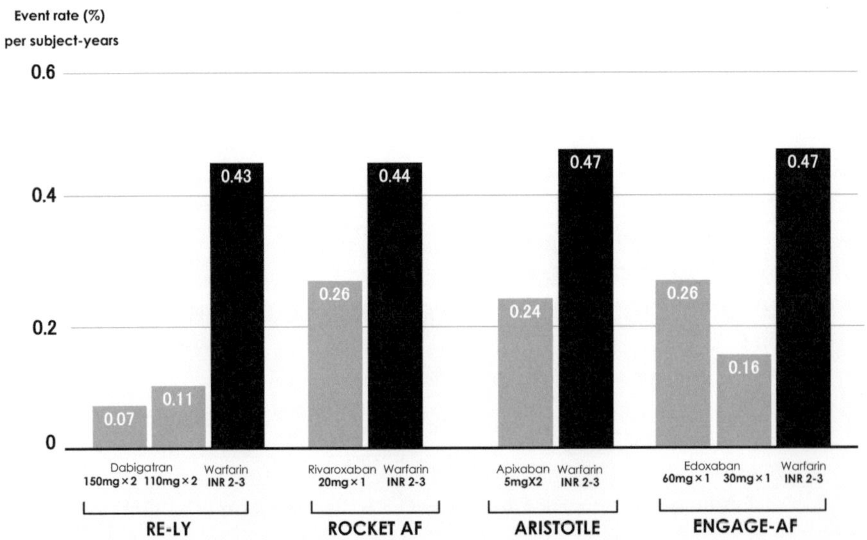

Fig. 3.4 Incidence of hemorrhagic stroke in phase III trials of NOACs.
The incidence of hemorrhagic stroke is based on the on-treatment analysis of each Phase III trial, quoted from Refs. [5–8]

with rivaroxaban (52.4 % vs. 76.8 %, $p < 0.008$) [20]. On the other hand, the proportion of subdural hematoma was lower with rivaroxaban than with dabigatran (14.6 % vs. 38.1 %, $p < 0.006$). Connolly et al. also reported that the risk of subdural hematoma with Xa inhibitors, but not with thrombin inhibitors, was similar to that with antiplatelet monotherapy [21]. Komori et al. retrospectively reviewed the clinical data and treatment summaries of nine intracranial bleeds that developed during dabigatran treatment in eight patients with non-valvular atrial fibrillation, and they found that only two episodes were intracerebral hemorrhage, and the other seven were trauma-related hemorrhage, including subdural hematoma [13].

This phenomenon observed in treatment with dabigatran may be due to not only the short half-life and maintained plasma level of VII but also the presence of thrombin-activatable fibrinolysis inhibitor (TAFI) and tissue factors rich in the brain, not outside the brain in the skull. Dabigatran interacts selectively and reversibly with the active site of the thrombin molecule, but it does not inhibit TAFI generation, leading to the downregulation of fibrinolysis [22–24]. Won et al. used dual-energy computed tomography in experimental mouse models of ICH treated with dabigatran or warfarin and found that dabigatran induced less extravasation of contrast medium, a marker of ongoing bleeding, than warfarin [23]. Lauer et al. demonstrated that, in contrast with warfarin, pretreatment with dabigatran did not increase hematoma volume in experimental mouse models of ICH [24].

3.4 East Asia vs. Non-East Asia

According to Phase III NOAC trials that compared (East) Asians with other populations, the former had a 20-kg lower body weight than Caucasians (an average of about 60–70 kg in the former and 80–90 kg in the latter) [9, 15, 17, 25–27]. When the body frame is small, kidney function is correlated with body weight, and thus (east) Asians have lower creatinine clearance than Caucasians. Among cardiovascular diseases, East Asians have a relatively lower incidence of myocardial infarction but a relatively higher incidence of cerebrovascular accidents than Caucasians [9, 15, 17, 25–27].

According to some epidemiological surveys, Japanese and other East Asians have a markedly higher incidence of intracranial hemorrhage than Westerners [28, 29]. One study in the USA that examined the incidence of intracranial hemorrhage during warfarin therapy showed that, compared to Caucasians, the incidence was twice as high among Hispanics and Blacks and as much as four times as high among Asians [30]. Some antithrombotic drugs show racial differences in the risk of major hemorrhage and intracranial hemorrhage. The concern that the incidence of such hemorrhage is higher in Japanese is reflected in the lower doses than in Western countries for alteplase in tPA thrombolytic therapy, the antiplatelet drug ticlopidine, and the Xa inhibitor rivaroxaban and also in the optimum dose management of warfarin. The causes of these racial differences are not clearly understood.

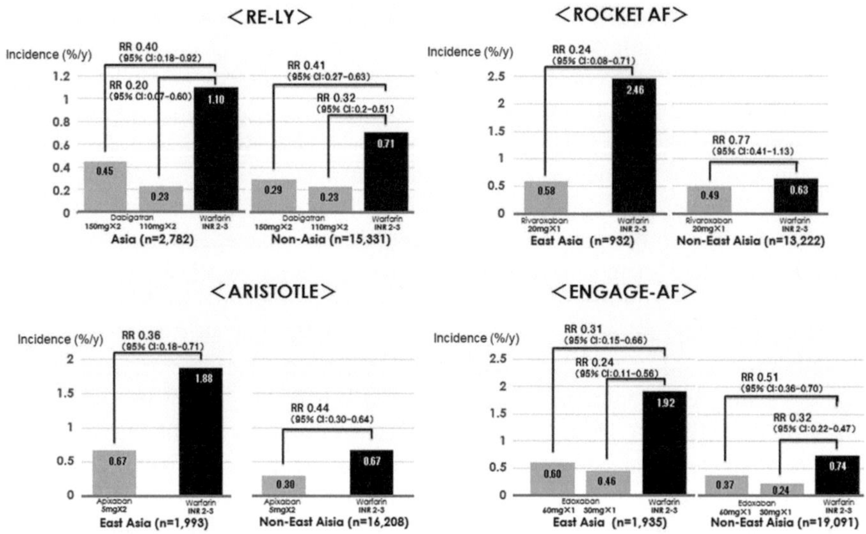

Fig. 3.5 Comparison of the incidence of intracranial hemorrhage between (East) Asians and Non-(East) Asians in NOAC trials.
The incidence of intracranial hemorrhage is much higher in (East) Asians than Non-(East) Asians with warfarin treatment. However, when an NOAC is used instead of warfarin, there is a significant reduction in the incidence of intracranial hemorrhage

Analysis of the results obtained for East Asians in Phase III trials showed that, though the warfarin dose was maintained at a lower level for East Asians, the incidence of intracranial hemorrhage was higher among East Asians than Caucasians [9, 15, 17, 25–27]. However, when an NOAC is used instead of warfarin, there is a significant reduction in the incidence of intracranial hemorrhage, to the level seen in Caucasians. Therefore, NOACs are expected to benefit all people but East Asians the most (Fig. 3.5).

3.5 Prevention

There are many risk factors predisposing to brain hemorrhage. Of them, control of blood pressure and blood sugar and cessation of smoking and excessive alcohol drinking are essential because they are risk factors that we can manage in the clinic.

The SPS3 study group investigated blood pressure targets in patients with recent lacunar stroke and secondary prevention using antiplatelets and found that a systolic blood pressure target of less than 130 mmHg was likely to be beneficial to avoid brain hemorrhage [31].

Toyoda et al. investigated the relationship between blood pressure levels and bleeding events during antithrombotic therapy in 4009 patients taking antiplatelets, anticoagulants, or both and found that the optimal cutoff blood pressure level to predict impending risk of intracranial hemorrhage was ≥130/81 mmHg [32].

3.6 Nonsurgical Measures

Although NOAC is superior to warfarin from standpoint of view of ICH, there are some reports regarding ICH during NOAC treatment with a poor prognosis. Shoji et al. reported five cases of intracranial hemorrhage related to dabigatran administration [33]. Outcomes were poor for all but one patient. Debata et al. reported three cases of ICH on rivaroxaban [34], with two patients showing fatal deterioration after admission, with hematoma expansion on CT. It seems quite important to understand the general measures required initially to prevent the expansion of intracerebral hematoma during NOAC treatment; the usefulness of charcoal administration to reduce NOAC absorption from the gastrointestinal tract; the application of hemodialysis to remove dabigatran [35]; the efficacy of coagulation factor therapy, including four-factor prothrombin complex concentrate and recombinant activated factor VII; and the need to develop antidotes for each NOAC (Table 3.2).

3.6.1 General Measures

In the event of an anticoagulant-associated major bleed, general measures are initially required [36–38]. First, to prevent any increase in the concentration of the anticoagulant, anticoagulants must be withheld. Second, if possible, active hemorrhage must be controlled by compressing or ligating the source of bleeding. Third, to maintain blood pressure within the normal range, lost fluids must be replaced using infusions of intravenous fluids so that the anticoagulant can be efficiently metabolized and excreted from the body; the half-life of NOACs is usually about a half a day. Fourth, if hemorrhagic stroke develops, systolic blood pressure needs to be kept under 140 mmHg [39].

Table 3.2 Hemostatic measures to reverse the anticoagulant effects of each NOAC

	Dabigatran	Rivaroxaban	Apixaban	Edoxaban
Oral activated charcoal	Yes	Yes	Yes	Yes
Hemodialysis	Yes	No	No	No
Four-factor PCC	Possible	Possible	Possible	Possible
Recombinant VIIa	Probably	Probably	Probably	Probably
Fresh frozen plasma	No	No	No	No

3.6.2 Four-Factor Prothrombin Complex Concentrate

Eerenberg et al. performed a randomized, double-blind, placebo-controlled study in which 12 healthy male volunteers received rivaroxaban 20 mg twice daily ($n = 6$) or dabigatran 150 mg twice daily ($n = 6$) for 2.5 days, followed by either a single bolus of 50 IU/kg four-factor PCC (Cofact) or a similar volume of saline [40]. After a washout period, this procedure was repeated with treatment with the other anticoagulant. Rivaroxaban induced a significant prolongation of the prothrombin time (15.8 ± 1.3 versus 12.3 ± 0.7 seconds at baseline; $P < 0.001$) that was immediately and completely reversed by PCC (12.8 ± 1.0; $P < 0.001$). The endogenous thrombin potential was inhibited by rivaroxaban (51 % ± 22%; baseline, 92 % ± 22%; $P < 0.002$) and normalized with PCC (114 % ± 26 %; P < 0.001), whereas saline had no effect. Dabigatran increased the activated partial thromboplastin time, ecarin clotting time, and thrombin time. Administration of PCC did not restore these coagulation results. It was concluded that PCC immediately and completely reverses the anticoagulant effect of rivaroxaban in healthy individuals, but it has no effect on the anticoagulant action of dabigatran, although bleeding was not evaluated in the participants.

Recently, the reversal of apixaban anticoagulation by four-factor PCCs in healthy subjects has been reported [41]. Perlstein et al. conducted an open-label, randomized, placebo-controlled, three-period crossover study in 15 healthy subjects administered with apixaban, 10 mg twice daily, for 3 days to attain steady-state concentrations. They received a 30-minute infusion of either 50-IU/kg Cofact or Beriplex or saline separately in three different periods. The study clearly demonstrated that both Cofact and Beriplex reversed the steady-state pharmacodynamic effects of apixaban in several coagulation assessments, including a thrombin generation assay. However, the efficacy of the four-factor PCCs on bleeding events in the subjects was not assessed.

Zahir et al. evaluated the effects of edoxaban (60 mg) on bleeding following punch biopsy and reversal by a four-factor PCC (Beriplex) in a double-blind, randomized, placebo-controlled, two-way crossover study in 110 healthy subjects and found that the four-factor PCC dose-dependently reversed the effects of edoxaban, with complete reversal of bleeding duration and endogenous thrombin potential and partial reversal of PT following intravenous administration of 50 IU/kg of four-factor PCC [42]. These results indicate that a four-factor PCC dose of 50 IU/kg is appropriate to reverse the effect of a therapeutic dose of edoxaban.

Hamada et al. reported a case of thalamic hemorrhage that occurred during anticoagulant therapy with rivaroxaban and expanded even after administration of PCC [43]. They found that administration of 1000 IU of PCC corrected prolonged PT-INR values immediately, but it did not correct anti-Xa activity, and they concluded that the anticoagulant effect of rivaroxaban may not be reversed by PCC or a greater amount of PCC may be required to reverse it.

3.6.3 Antidotes

There are three potential antidotes for NOAC in development, idarucizumab, andexanet alfa, and ciraparantag (arapazine) (Table 3.3).

3.6.3.1 Idarucizumab

Idarucizumab is a dabigatran-specific reversal agent, a fully humanized mouse monoclonal antibody fragment (Fab) [44, 45]. It seems that the binding pattern of the Fab is similar to the binding pattern of dabigatran to thrombin. The affinity of the Fab for thrombin is 350 times stronger than that of dabigatran, and the Fab has no effect on coagulation or platelet activity. Pollack et al. performed a prospective cohort study to determine the safety of 5 g of intravenous idarucizumab and its capacity to reverse the anticoagulant effects of dabigatran in 90 patients who had serious bleeding or required an urgent procedure, and they concluded that idarucizumab completely reversed the anticoagulant effect of dabigatran within minutes [46] (Fig. 3.6). The US Food and Drug Administration (FDA) granted approval of idarucizumab for patients treated with dabigatran, when reversal of the anticoagulant effects of dabigatran was needed for emergency surgery/urgent procedures or in life-threatening or uncontrolled bleeding.

Table 3.3 Antidotes

	Idarucizumab (BI 655075) aDabi-Fab	Andexanet alfa (PRT064445, or PRT4445)	Ciraparantag (Arapazine, PER977)
Company	Boehringer Ingelheim	Portola	
Characteristics	Monoclonal antibody/Fab	Recombinant factor Xa decoy	
Administration	Intravenous	Intravenous	
Subjects of anticoagulants	Dabigatran	Rivaroxaban	Dabigatran
		Apixaban	Rivaroxaban
		Edoxaban	Apixaban
		LMWH	Edoxaban
			LMWH
			UFH
Stage of development	Phase III	Phase III for rivaroxaban and apixaban	Phase II~III for edoxaban

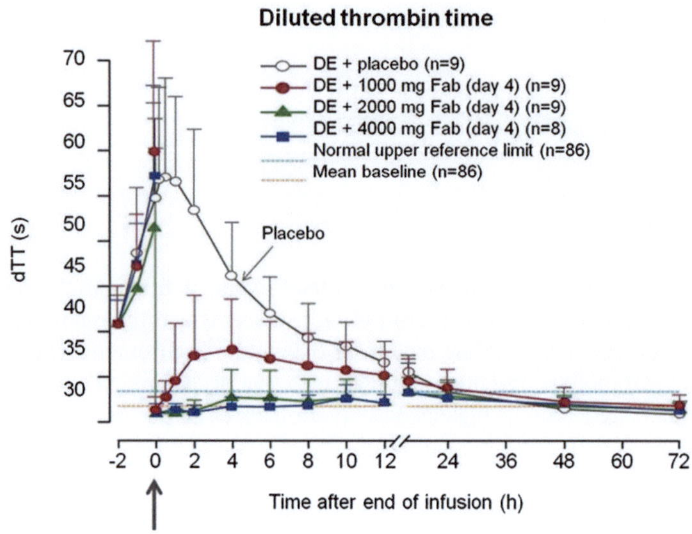

Fig. 3.6 Reversal of dabigatran-induced anticoagulation with antibody fragment (Fab), measured by diluted thrombin time. *dTT* diluted thrombin time, *DE* dabigatran etexilate. *Arrow*: starting administration of antibody (Fab). Image: Boehringer Ingelheim GmbH from http://www.boehringer-ingelheim.com/news/news_releases/press_releases/2013/18_november_2013dabigatranetexilate.html

3.6.3.2 Andexanet Alfa

Andexanet alfa is a recombinant, human coagulation factor Xa decoy that is produced in Chinese hamster ovary cells [44, 45, 47]. It is similar to native factor Xa but lacks the gamma-carboxyglutamic acid domain required for efficient incorporation into the thrombinase complex. It has the ability to bind to the factor Xa inhibitors, rivaroxaban, apixaban, and edoxaban, and to reverse their anticoagulant effects. The Phase III study of randomized trial for andexanet alfa demonstrated that it reversed the anticoagulant activity of apixaban and rivaroxaban in older healthy participants within minutes after administration and for the duration of infusion, without evidence of clinical toxic effects [48]. The development for edoxaban was also started.

3.6.3.3 Ciraparantag (Arapazine)

Ciraparantag (Arapazine, PER977) is a small, synthetic, water-soluble molecular substance directly binding with unfractionated heparin, low-molecular-weight heparin, dabigatran, rivaroxaban, apixaban, and edoxaban, and it reverses their anticoagulant effects through noncovalent hydrogen bonding and charge-charge interactions [45, 49]. In edoxaban-treated healthy volunteers, it decreased clotting times [49].

References

1. Yasaka M, Minematsu K, Naritomi H, Sakata T, Yamaguchi T. Predisposing factors for enlargement of intracerebral hemorrhage in patients treated with warfarin. Thromb Haemost. 2003;89:2782–3.
2. Itabashi R, Yasaka M, Kuwashiro T, Nakagaki H, Miyashita F, Naritomi H, et al. Location of acute brain hemorrhage in patients undergoing antithrombotic therapy. J Neurol Sci. 2009;280:87–9.
3. Toyoda K, Yasaka M, Nagata K, Nagao T, Gotoh J, Sakamoto T, et al. Antithrombotic therapy influences location, enlargement, and mortality from intracerebral hemorrhage. The Bleeding with Antithrombotic Therapy (BAT) Retrospective Study. Cerebrovasc Dis. 2009;27:151–9.
4. Kuwashiro T, Yasaka M, Itabashi R, Nakagaki H, Miyashita F, Naritomi H, et al. Enlargement of acute intracerebral hematomas in patients on long-term warfarin treatment. Cerebrovasc Dis. 2010;29:446–53.
5. Connolly SJ, Ezekowitz MD, Yusuf S, Eikelboom J, Oldgren J, Parekh A, et al. RE-LY Steering Committee and Investigators: dabigatran versus warfarin in patients with atrial fibrillation. N Engl J Med. 2009;361:1139–51 and Erratum in: N Engl J Med. 2010; 363:1877.
6. Patel MR, Mahaffey KW, Garg J, Pan G, Singer DE, Hacke W, The ROCKET AF Investigators, et al. Rivaroxaban versus warfarin in nonvalvular atrial fibrillation. N Engl J Med. 2011;365:883–91.
7. Granger CB, Alexander JH, McMurray JJ, Lopes RD, Hylek EM, Hanna M, ARISTOTLE Committees and Investigators, et al. . Apixaban versus warfarin in patients with atrial fibrillation. N Engl J Med. 2011;365:981–92.
8. Giugliano RP, Ruff CT, Braunwald E, Murphy SA, Wiviott SD, Halperin JL, et al. Edoxaban versus warfarin in patients with atrial fibrillation. N Engl J Med. 2013;369:2093–104
9. Hori M, Matsumoto M, Tanahashi N, Momomura S, Uchiyama S, Goto S, et al. Rivaroxaban vs. warfarin in Japanese patients with atrial fibrillation – the J-ROCKET AF study . Circ J. 2012;76:2104–11.
10. Hart RG, Diener HC, Yang S, Connolly SJ, Wallentin L, Reilly PA, et al. Intracranial hemorrhage in atrial fibrillation patients during anticoagulation with warfarin or dabigatran: The RE-LY trial. Stroke. 2012;43:1511–7.
11. Graham DJ, Reichman MF, Wernecke M, Zhang R, Southworth MR, Levenson M, et al. Cardiovascular, bleeding, and mortality risks in elderly Medicare patients treated with dabigatran or warfarin for non-valvular atrial fibrillation. Circulation. 2015;131:157–64.
12. Hagii J, Tomita H, Metoki N, Saito S, Shiroto H, Hitomi H, et al. Characteristics of intracerebral hemorrhage during rivaroxaban treatment: comparison with those during warfarin. Stroke. 2014;45:2805–7.
13. Komori M, Yasaka M, Kokuba K, Matsuoka H, Fujimoto S, Yoshida M, et al. Intracranial hemorrhage during dabigatran treatment. Circ J. 2014;78:1335–41.
14. Hylek EM, Held C, Alexander JH, Lopes RD, De Caterina R, et al. Major bleeding in patients with atrial fibrillation receiving apixaban or warfarin: the ARISTOTLE Trial (Apixaban for Reduction in Stroke and Other Thromboembolic Events in Atrial Fibrillation): predictors, characteristics, and clinical outcomes. J Am Coll Cardiol. 2014;63:2141–7.
15. Yasaka M. J-ROCKET AF trial increased expectation of lower-dose rivaroxaban made for Japan. Circ J. 2012;76:2086–7.
16. Wong KS, Hu D, Oomman A, Tan RS, Patel M, Singer D, et al. Rivaroxaban for stroke prevention in East Asia patients from the ROCKET AF trial. Stroke. 2014;45:1739–49.
17. Yasaka M, Lip GY. Stroke prevention in Asian patients with atrial fibrillation. Stroke. 2014;45:1608–9.
18. Ohmura T, Ikegami K, Hori K, Encinas J, Maruyama I. Effect of anticoagulant drug dabigatran etexilate on thrombus formation and bleeding in an AV shunted model and effect of vitamin K on the antithrombotic action. Pharma Medica. 2011;29:137–42.

19. Yasaka M. New insights into nonvitamin K antagonist oral anticoagulants' reversal of intracerebral hemorrhage. Front Neurol Neurosci. 2015;37:93–106.
20. Saji N, Kimura K, Aoki J, Uemura J, Sakamoto Y. Intracranial hemorrhage caused by Non-Vitamin K Antagonist Oral Anticoagulants (NOACs). Multicenter retrospective cohort study in Japan. Circ J. 2015;79:1018–23.
21. Connolly BJ, Pearce LA, Hart RG. Vitamin K antagonists and risk of subdural hematoma: meta-analysis of randomized clinical trials. Stroke. 2014;45:1672–8.
22. Hirano T. New era of oral anticoagulation for Japanese non-valvular atrial fibrillation patients. Circ J. 2014;78:1317–9.
23. Won SY, Schlunk F, Dinkel J, Karatas H, Leung W, Hayakawa K, et al. Imaging of contrast medium extravasation in anticoagulation-associated intracerebral hemorrhage with dual-energy computed tomography. Stroke. 2013;44:2883–90.
24. Lauer A, Cianchetti FA, Van Cott EM, Schlunk F, Schulz E, Pfeilschifter W, et al. Anticoagulation with the oral direct thrombin inhibitor dabigatran does not enlarge hematoma volume in experimental intracerebral hemorrhage. Circulation. 2011;124:1654–62.
25. Wong KS, Hu DY, Oomman A, Tan RS, Patel MR, Singer DE, et al. Rivaroxaban for stroke prevention in East Asia patients from the ROCKET AF trial. Stroke. 2014;45:1739–47.
26. Goto S, Zhu J, Liu L, Oh BH, Wojdyla DM, Aylward P, et al. Efficacy and safety of apixaban compared with warfarin for stroke prevention in patients with atrial fibrillation from East Asia: a sub-analysis of the 50 literature cited apixaban for reduction in stroke and other thromboembolic events in atrial fibrillation(ARISTOTLE) trial. AHJ. 2014;168:303–9.
27. Yamashita T, Koretsune Y, Yang Y, Chen SA, Chung N, Shimada YJ, et al. Edoxaban vs. warfarin in East Asian patients with atrial fibrillation: an ENGAGE AF-TIMI 48 subanalysis. Circ J. 2016;80:860–9.
28. Toyoda K. Problems concerning antithrombotic therapy for Japanese patients: lessons from the Bleeding with Antithrombotic Therapy (BAT) study. J Jpn Soc Thromb Hemost. 2009;20:594–601.
29. van Asch CJ, Luitse MJ, Rinkel GJ, van der Tweel I, Algra A, Klijn CJ. Incidence, case fatality, and functional outcome of intracerebral haemorrhage over time, according to age, sex, and ethnic origin: a systematic review and meta-analysis. Lancet Neurol. 2010;9:167–76.
30. Shen AY, Yao JF, Brar SS, Jorgensen MB, Chen W. Racial/ethnic differences in the risk of intracranial hemorrhage among patients with atrial fibrillation. J Am Coll Cardiol. 2007;50:309–15.
31. Benavente OR, Coffey CS, Conwit R, Hart RG, McClure LA, Pearce LA, et al. Blood-pressure targets in patients with recent lacunar stroke: the SPS3 randomised trial. Lancet. 2013;382:507–15.
32. Toyoda K, Yasaka M, Uchiyama S, Nagao T, Gotoh J, Nagata K, et al. Blood pressure levels and bleeding events during antithrombotic therapy: the Bleeding with Antithrombotic Therapy (BAT) Study. Stroke. 2010;41:1440–4.
33. Shoji A, Satoh K, Nakano Y, Sumitomo H, Niki H, et al. Dabigatran related intracranial hemorrhage, five cases report. Jpn J Stroke. 2014;36:186–90 (Abstract with English).
34. Debata A, Tateishi Y, Hamabe J, Horie N, Izumo T, Hayashi K, et al. Three cases of spontaneous intracerebral hemorrhage under rivaroxaban. Jpn J Stroke. 2015; in press (Abstract with English).
35. Singh T, Maw TT, Henry BL, Pastor-Soler NM, Unruh ML, Hallows KR, et al. Extracorporeal therapy for dabigatran removal in the treatment of acute bleeding: a single center experience. Clin J Am Soc Nephurol. 2013;8:1533–9.
36. Kaatz S, Kouides PA, Garcia DA, Spyropolous AC, Crowther M, Douketis JD, et al. Guidance on the emergent reversal of oral thrombin and factor Xa inhibitors. Am J Hematol. 2012;87(Suppl 1):S141–5.
37. Hankey GJ. Unanswered questions and research priorities to optimise stroke prevention in atrial fibrillation with the new oral anticoagulants. Thromb Haemost. 2014;111:808–16.

38. Miller MP, Trujillo TC, Nordenholz KE. Practical considerations in emergency management of bleeding in the setting of target-specific oral anticoagulants. Am J Emerg Med. 2014;32:375–82.
39. Anderson CS, Huang Y, Wang JG, Arima H, Neal B, Peng B, et al. Intensive blood pressure reduction in acute cerebral haemorrhage trial (INTERACT): a randomised pilot trial. Lancet Neurol. 2008;7:391–9.
40. Eerenberg ES, Kamphuisen PW, Sijpkens MK, Meijers JC, Buller HR, Levi M. Reversal of rivaroxaban and dabigatran by prothrombin complex concentrate. a randomized, placebo-controlled, crossover study in healthy subjects. Circulation. 2011;124:1573–9
41. Perlstein I, Wang Z, Yan Song Y, et al.: Reversal of apixaban anticoagulation by 4-factor prothrombin complex concentrates in healthy subjects. 56th Americal Society of Hematology Annual Meeting and Exposition, San Francisco, December, 2014
42. Zahir H1, Brown KS2, Vandell AG2, Desai M2, Maa JF2, Dishy V, et al.: Edoxaban effects on bleeding following punch biopsy and reversal by a 4-factor prothrombin complex concentrate. Circulation. 2015; 131:82-90
43. Hamada H, Wasa S, Mima Y, Yasaka M, Kuwashiro T, Okada Y. A case of thalamic hemorrhage which occurred during anticoagulant therapy with Xa inhibitor and expanded even after the administration of ptorhrombin complex concentrate. Jpn Stroke J. 2016; in press.
44. Vanden Daelen S, Peetermans M, Vanassche T, Verhamme P, Vandermeulen E. Monitoring and reversal strategies for new oral anticoagulants. Expert Rev Cardiovasc Ther. 2015;13:95–103.
45. Costin J, Ansell J, Laulicht B, Bakhru S, Steiner S. Reversal agents in development for the new oral anticoagulants. Postgrad Med. 2014;126:19–24.
46. Pollack Jr CV, Reilly PA, Eikelboom J, Glund S, Verhamme P, Bernstein RA, et al. Idarucizumab for dabigatran reversal. N Engl J Med. 2015;373:511–20.
47. Lu G, DeGuzman FR, Hollenbach SJ, Karbarz MJ, Abe K, Lee G, et al. A specific antidote for reversal of anticoagulation by direct and indirect inhibitors of coagulation factor Xa. Nat Med. 2013;19:446–51.
48. Siegal DM, Curnutte JT, Connolly SJ, Lu G, Conley PB, Wiens BL, et al. Andexanet alfa for the reversal of factor Xa inhibitor activity. N Engl J Med. 2015;373:2413–24.
49. Ansell JE1, Bakhru SH, Laulicht BE, Steiner SS, Grosso M, Brown K, et al.: Use of PER977 to reverse the anticoagulant effect of edoxaban. N Engl J Med. 2014;371:2141-2142.

Chapter 4
Severity and Outcomes of Intracerebral Bleeding and Cardiac Cerebral Embolism

Hirofumi Tomita, Joji Hagii, and Ken Okumura

Abstract Although it is of significant interest and importance for clinical practice to evaluate stroke severity and functional outcome in patients with intracerebral bleeding (ICH) and cardiac cerebral embolism (CCE) occurring during non-vitamin K antagonist oral anticoagulants (NOACs) treatment, clinical research addressing these critical issues in a real-world setting is limited. In this chapter, we discuss these issues by comparing the outcomes of ICH and CCE occurring during warfarin treatment. We and others showed that NOAC-associated ICH may occur in patients at high risk of bleeding events and that even if ICH occurs during NOAC treatment, the size of hematoma is relatively small and hematoma expansion occurs less frequently compared with warfarin-associated ICH. Involvement of microbleeds in NOAC-associated ICH and possible underlying mechanisms for favorable outcome of NOAC-associated ICH are still under investigation. On the other hand, there are some reports in the opposite direction showing hematoma expansion and poor clinical outcomes in patients with ICH occurring during NOAC treatment. More studies are warranted. CCE occurring during NOAC treatment was associated with a reduced stroke severity on admission and a favorable functional outcome at discharge, similarly to that during warfarin treatment at a therapeutic range. However, discontinuation of NOAC or its temporary interruption is possibly associated with poor outcome. Therefore, adherence to NOAC and its management is considerably important.

Keywords NOAC • Intracerebral bleeding • Cerebral embolism • Stroke severity • Modified Rankin Scale

---

H. Tomita, M.D. (✉)
Department of Cardiology, Hirosaki University Graduate School of Medicine, 5 Zaifu-cho, Hirosaki 036-8562, Japan

Department of Hypertension and Stroke Medicine, Hirosaki University Graduate School of Medicine, 5 Zaifu-cho, Hirosaki 036-8562, Japan
e-mail: tomitah@hirosaki-u.ac.jp

J. Hagii, M.D.
Hirosaki Stroke and Rehabilitation Center, 1-2-1 Ougimachi, Hirosaki 036-8104, Japan

K. Okumura, M.D.
Advanced Arrhythmia Therapeutic Branch, Division of Cardiology, Saiseikai Kumamoto Hospital, 5-3-1 Chikami, Minami-ku, Kumamoto 861-4193, Japan

M. Uno, K. Ogasawara (eds.), *Treatment of Non-vitamin K Antagonist Oral Anticoagulants*, DOI 10.1007/978-981-10-1878-7_4

4.1 Introduction

Non-vitamin K antagonist oral anticoagulants (NOACs) including dabigatran, rivaroxaban, apixaban, and edoxaban have been widely used for the prevention of stroke and systemic thromboembolism in patients with nonvalvular atrial fibrillation (NVAF) [1–4]. A meta-analysis including the four phase III clinical trials, RE-LY, ROCKET-AF, ARISTOTLE, and ENGAGE AF-TIMI 48 trials, demonstrated a favorable outcome with significant reductions in stroke, intracranial hemorrhage (ICH), and all-cause mortality and a similar major bleeding risk to warfarin [5]. In addition to this favorable profile of NOACs, it is of significant interest and importance for clinical practice to evaluate stroke severity and functional outcome in patients with ICH and cardiac cerebral embolism (CCE) occurring during NOAC treatment. However, there has been few clinical research addressing these critical issues in a real-world setting.

In this chapter, we describe an outline of stroke severity and functional outcomes of patients with ICH and CE occurring during NOAC treatment by comparing those during warfarin treatment.

4.2 Intracerebral Hemorrhage During NOAC Treatment

4.2.1 Severity and Outcome of Intracerebral Hemorrhage

Numerous studies showed hematoma expansion and poor clinical outcomes in patients with ICH occurring during warfarin therapy [6]. Furthermore, using the data from the consecutive 870 ICH patients (mean 68 ± 13 years) admitted to the Hirosaki Stroke and Rehabilitation Center (HSRC), we recently showed that mean prothrombin time-international normalized ratio (PT-INR) within 24 h after the onset of ICH in patients with warfarin treatment was 2.27 ± 0.62 ($n = 65$), and 56 of them (86 %) showed PT-INR < 2.8 [7]. This finding indicates that ICH occurs not necessarily in patients with warfarin overdose but rather in those with PT-INR levels within the therapeutic range.

In the last few years, reports have been accumulating on the NOAC-associated ICH. We first reported a real-world evidence on stroke severity and functional outcome in patients with ICH that occurred during NOAC treatment [8]. Of 585 patients with ICH admitted to the HSRC from April 2011 through October 2013, 5 patients had ICH occurring during rivaroxaban treatment and 56 during warfarin treatment. Clinical characteristics of the patients between the two groups were compared. There were no differences in mean age, $CHADS_2$ and HAS-BLED scores, renal function, and antiplatelet use between the two groups, whereas a past history of ICH was found more in patients with rivaroxaban than in those with warfarin (3/5, 60 % versus 7/56, 13 %, $p = 0.03$). All five patients with rivaroxaban treatment had HAS-BLED score of 3 before admission. Patients with rivaroxaban had markedly small hematoma volumes compared with those with warfarin (median 4 (interquartile range 2–5) versus 11 (7–34) mL, $p = 0.02$), and hematoma volume was ≤10 mL in all rivaroxaban patients. None of the patients with rivaroxaban showed hematoma expansion after admission and underwent surgical treatment. In contrast, of the patients with warfarin, ten (18 %) showed hematoma expansion, and six (11 %) underwent surgical treatment for its removal. These findings suggest that although ICH occurs also in patients taking rivaroxaban, especially at high risk of major bleeding, the influence of rivaroxaban to hematoma volume and enlargement seems to be smaller than that of warfarin. Representative radiographical images of ICH occurring during warfarin and rivaroxaban treatments are shown in Figs. 4.1 and 4.2, respectively.

We also investigated the clinical outcomes of the patients with ICH occurring during rivaroxaban and warfarin treatments. When the patients with modified Rankin Scale (mRS) ≤1 before admission were analyzed, none of those with rivaroxaban showed mRS >4 at discharge, whereas almost a half of those with warfarin showed mRS >4 at discharge. Furthermore, none of the patients with rivaroxaban died during hospitalization, whereas ten patients (18 %) with warfarin died. These findings indicate that patients with ICH during rivaroxaban treatment had favorable stroke severity and functional outcomes compared with those during warfarin treatment.

Recent reports from the Japanese investigators also support our findings [9–11]. Case series of eight patients with intracranial hemorrhage during dabigatran treatment, an oral direct thrombin inhibitor, showed that the hematoma caused by acute intracranial bleedings, including five chronic subdural hematomas (SDHs), two ICHs, and one traumatic subarachnoid hemorrhage (SAH), remained small or mod-

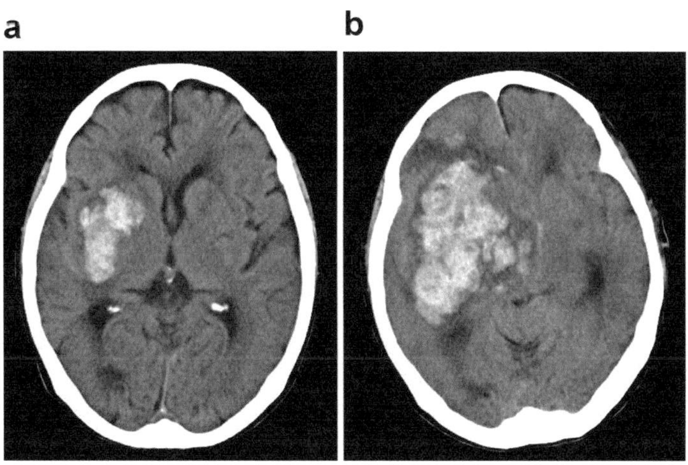

Fig. 4.1 Representative computed tomography (*CT*) in a patient with intracerebral hemorrhage occurring during warfarin treatment
CT images at admission (**a**) and after 1 h (**b**) are shown. Expansion of hematoma was observed 1 h after the admission

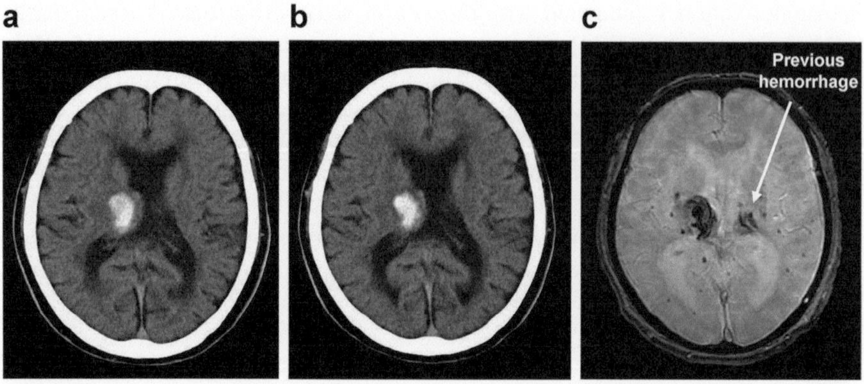

Fig. 4.2 Representative computed tomography (CT) and T2*-weighted magnetic resonance imaging (MRI) in a patient with intracerebral hemorrhage occurring during rivaroxaban treatment
CT images at admission (Day 1) (**a**) and at day 4 (**b**), and T2*-weighted MRI at day 4 (**c**) are shown. No expansion of hematoma was observed. *Arrow* indicates previous hemorrhage. Multiple cerebral microbleeds were observed (Copyright permission was obtained from the publisher of the article [8])

erate and did not expand [9]. Saji et al. performed a nationwide anonymous questionnaire survey to investigate the clinical outcomes of NOAC-associated ICH in Japan. The results showed that the incidence of NOAC-associated ICH appears to be low and patients with NOAC-associated ICH have low incidences of hematoma enlargement and mortality [10]. Akiyama et al. further reported radiographical analyses of six NOAC-associated ICHs (five rivaroxaban and one dabigatran). They found that the hematoma volume of NOAC-associated ICH was small and did not expand even in the absence of infusion of reversal agents [11].

More recently, Wilson et al. reported similar results in multicenter prospective observational study performed in the UK [12]. They compared clinical outcomes between 11 patients with NOAC-associated ICH and 52 with warfarin-associated ICH. The results showed that the median hematoma volume was 2.4 (0.3–5.4) mL in patients with NOAC-associated ICH and 8.9 (4.0–21.3) mL in those with warfarin-associated ICH ($p = 0.003$). Ordinal logistic regression analysis further showed increased odds ratio of a worse outcome in warfarin-associated ICH compared with NOAC-associated ICH (odds ratio (OR) 4.46, 95 % confidence interval (CI) 1.10–18.14, $p = 0.037$). Furthermore, a recent sub-analysis of the ARISTOTLE study showed that mortality ratio at 30 days after major bleeding events was lower by 50 % in patients randomized to apixaban than in those to warfarin [13]. The pooled data analysis including the RE-LY study showed that the 30-day mortality after the first major bleeding events tended to be lower in patients with dabigatran (9.1 %) than in those with warfarin (13.0 %) (OR, 0.68, 95 % CI, 0.46–1.01, $P = 0.057$). After adjusting confounders, OR for 30-day mortality with dabigatran versus warfarin was 0.66 (95%CI 0.44–1.00, $p = 0.051$) [14].

Taken together, all these reports including ours indicate that NOAC-associated ICH may occur in patients at high risk of bleeding events, but even if ICH occurs during NOAC treatment, the size of hematoma is relatively small and hematoma expansion occurs less frequently. These may lead to potential benefits for stroke severity and functional outcome in NOAC-associated ICH.

On the other hand, there are some reports in the opposite direction showing hematoma expansion and poor clinical outcomes in patients with ICH occurring during NOAC treatment [15–18]. Case reports showed that secondary hematoma expansion occurred in ICH patient during rivaroxaban [15] and dabigatran treatment [16]. Beynon et al. also analyzed clinical outcomes of 55 patients with NOAC-associated ICH (42 rivaroxaban, 7 apixaban, and 6 dabigatran) caused by 18 traumatic SAH/ICH, 24 acute or chronic SDH, 1 spontaneous SAH, and 10 spontaneous ICH in a single-center retrospective study performed in Germany [17]. They reported that the 30-day mortality was 20 % and renal impairment was involved in this increased mortality. More recently, Purrucker et al. reported early clinical and radiological course and outcome of 61 patients (mean age 76.1 years, median CHA_2DS_2-VAS_C = 5, median HAS-BLED = 2) with NOAC-associated nontraumatic ICH (49 rivaroxaban, 5 apixaban, and 7 dabigatran) in multicenter prospective observational study performed in Germany [18]. They found that mean hematoma volume was 23.7 (SD = 31.3) mL and hematoma expansion occurred in 38 %. Overall mortality was 28 % at 3 months and 65 % (17 of 45) of survivors had an unfavorable outcome (mRS 3–6). It should be pointed out that in these recent reports, the severity and outcome of NOAC-associated ICH were not compared with those of warfarin-associated ICH. Furthermore, the sub-analysis of the ROCKET-AF study showed that similar fatality rates on ICH were observed between rivaroxaban and warfarin (48 % versus 50 %), although radiographic analyses were not provided in the study [19].

Thus, there is a discrepancy in radiological and clinical outcome of NOAC-associated ICH among the studies. Differences in clinical backgrounds of patients, therapy after hospitalization, study design, and others may influence to the results. Further clinical studies are warranted to accumulate evidences regarding hematoma volume, hematoma expansion, and clinical outcomes in patients with NOAC-associated ICH.

4.2.2 *Potential Involvement of Cerebral Microbleeds*

Cerebral microbleeds (CMBs) are small, round low-intensity lesions detected in T2*-weighted or gradient-recall echo magnetic resonance imaging (MRI). Recent meta-analysis showed that the presence of CMBs is associated with an increased risk of future ICH, particularly in the Asian population [20]. Furthermore, an excess of CMBs is more frequent in ICH patients during warfarin treatment compared with those without warfarin [21]. These findings indicate that the presence of CMBs can be a useful predictive neuroradiological marker for ICH in warfarin-treated Asian population. Moreover, the presence of CMBs has been shown to be an independent risk factor for large-sized hemorrhage [22]. Thus, a considerable interest has been shown in the association between CMBs and subsequent ICH in patients treated with NOAC (12). We recently showed that multiple CMBs (CMBs >4) were detected more frequently in patients with rivaroxaban than in those with warfarin (4/5, 80 % versus 12/42, 29 %, $p = 0.04$). Representative CT images and T2*-weighted MRI in a patient with rivaroxaban treatment are shown in Fig. 4.2c.

Several multicenter prospective cohort studies including the Clinical Relevance of Microbleeds in Stroke (CROMIS-2) and the Cerebral Microbleeds as Predictor of Future Intra-Cerebral Hemorrhage During NOACs or Warfarin Therapy in NVAF Patients With Acute Ischemic Stroke (CMB-NOW) have been proposed to address the relationship between the presence of CMBs and anticoagulant-associated ICH [23, 24]. Results of these studies are awaited with great interest.

4.2.3 Potential Mechanisms for Favorable Outcome of NOAC-Associated ICH

Though not conclusive, we would introduce potential mechanisms for the favorable outcome of NOAC-associated ICH compared to that of warfarin-associated ICH. Warfarin inhibits multiple coagulation factors (II, VII, IX, and X) and regulatory factors protein C and S, whereas NOACs suppress only a single coagulation factor Xa or thrombin. The difference in half-time between warfarin and NOACs may also affect hematoma volume and expansion, 36–42 h in warfarin and 5–15 h in NOACs [25]. Warfarin exerts its effect through 24 h, whereas NOACs inhibit a target molecule in a concentration-dependent manner after taking, namely, they have a trough and peak cycle every 12 or 24 h. The formation of the tissue factor-factor VIIa complexes is an important initial step for coagulation cascade. Tissue factor is at high concentration in the brain and thereby plays an important role in the hemostatic system after ICH. Warfarin inhibits coagulation factor VII, which leads to lower formation of tissue factor and VIIa complex, whereas NOACs do not inhibit this process. All above differences in actions between warfarin and NOACs may explain the different outcomes of NOAC-associated and warfarin-associated ICH.

Furthermore, it may be of interest to investigate thrombin generation, since excess thrombin generation generally tends to be toward thrombosis and lack of generation toward bleeding events. As a half-time of thrombin is very short, it is difficult to measure quantity of thrombin accurately. Factor Xa converts prothrombin to thrombin, which leads to the conversion of fibrinogen to fibrin followed by clot formation. When one thrombin is produced by factor Xa during this process, one prothrombin fragment 1 + 2 (F1 + 2) molecule is generated. Therefore, plasma F1 + 2 measurement is inferred to be a sensitive marker of thrombin generation. Plasma F1 + 2 levels are shown to be decreased below the normal range in patients with warfarin treatment even if it is within therapeutic range [26]. In this context, it is of great interest to investigate effects of NOACs on plasma F1 + 2 levels or thrombin generation. Further clinical and experimental studies in this regard are warranted.

4.3 Cardiac Cerebral Embolism During NOAC Treatment

4.3.1 Severity and Outcome of Cardiac Cerebral Embolism

Efficacy of warfarin at therapeutic range for stroke prevention is well established [27]. On the contrary, poorly controlled warfarin does not decrease the risk of stroke in AF patients [28]. Indeed, using the data from the consecutive 846 CCE patients (mean 78 ± 9 years) admitted to the HSRC, we recently showed that mean PT-INR within 24 h after the CCE onset in NVAF patients treated with warfarin was 1.34 ± 0.33 (n = 129), and 111 of them (86 %) showed PT-INR values below the recommended therapeutic range in Japan [7], indicating poor warfarin control in most of the patients with CCE occurring during warfarin treatment. Furthermore, CCE patients with warfarin treatment at therapeutic range on admission are shown to have a reduced stroke severity and favorable functional outcome at discharge compared with those at lower range [27, 29]. These findings indicate that patients with well-controlled warfarin have not only a reduced incidence of CCE but a favorable functional outcome compared with those with poor warfarin control.

We recently showed that stroke severity and functional outcome of the patients with CCE occurred during NOAC treatment in comparison with those during warfarin treatment and with no anticoagulants in a real-world population [30]. Of 644 patients with CCE admitted to the HSRC from April 2011 through March 2014, 355 CCE patients within 48 h after the onset and with mRS ≤1 before the onset were analyzed. Of them, 262 patients (74 %) were treated with no anticoagulants (non-AC group), 63 (18 %) with warfarin below therapeutic range recommended in Japan (PT-INR < 1.6, WF-Lo group), 16 (5 %) with warfarin within therapeutic range (PT-INR ≥ 1.6, WF-Tp group), and 14 (4 %) with NOACs (9 dabigatran and 5 rivaroxaban, NOAC-DR group) before the onset of stroke. Clinical characteristics, stroke severity on admission, and functional outcome at discharge were compared among the four groups, non-AC, WF-Lo, WF-Tp, and NOAC-DR groups. All patient groups showed high $CHADS_2$ score (median, 3) and CHA_2DS_2-VASc score (median, 5), indicating high-risk patients for thromboembolism included. Stroke severity was assessed by the National Institutes of Health Stroke Scale (NIHSS) score on admission. The patients in the WF-Tp and NOAC-DR groups had lower NIHSS scores than those in the non-AC and WF-Lo groups (median, 5 (1–15) and 5 (3–6) versus 11 (5–19) and 12 (5–19), respectively) (Fig. 4.3). The patients in the WF-Tp and NOAC-DR groups also had a favorable functional outcome at discharge compared with those in the non-AC and WF-Lo groups (median mRS, 1 (0–4) and 1 (1–2) versus 2 (1–4) and 3 (1–5), respectively) (Fig. 4.4). More than 60 % of the patients with the WF-Tp and NOAC-DR groups have a favorable functional outcome (mRS 0 and 1) at discharge, whereas only 30 % of the patients with the non-AC and WF-Lo groups have a favorable one (Fig. 4.4). These findings indicate that CCE patients with NOAC treatment had a reduced stroke severity on admission and favorable functional outcome at discharge, similarly to those with warfarin treatment at therapeutic range. As there are very few clinical papers addressing this important issue, more evidence should be accumulated.

A potential mechanism by which CCE patients with NOAC treatment have a favorable outcome remains unclear. Varin et al. recently showed that rivaroxaban is likely to form a looser fibrin clot [31]. Further studies aimed at unraveling its mechanism are awaited with great interest.

4.3.2 Importance of Adherence to NOAC

Drug adherence is an important clinical issue. Recent paper showed that poor adherence to dabigatran was associated with an increased risk for stroke and all-cause mortality [32]. We also showed that, of the 14 CCE patients with NOAC treatment, 4 were poorly adherent, such as irregular intake of NOAC (1 dabigatran and 3 rivaroxaban), and 4 had a temporary interruption due to gastrointestinal endoscopic procedure, finger surgery, or worsened renal function prior to the stroke onset (all dabigatran) [30]. Notably, 2 patients in the NOAC-DR group, who had high NIHSS score (22 and 27) (Fig. 4.3) on admission and high mRS at discharge (5 and 6) (Fig. 4.4), had a temporary interruption of dabigatran. Consistent with this finding, Hayashi et al. reported stroke severity and functional outcome in 15 patients with NVAF-associated ischemic stroke treated with dabigatran. Nine patients had a regular taking of the drug (treatment group), whereas six had discontinued (discontinuation group) [33]. The comparison between the two groups showed that patients with the discontinuation group had a significantly higher NIHSS score on admission and poor functional outcome at discharge compared with those with the treatment group (median 12.5 (1–19) versus 1 (1–5) for NIHSS, $p = 0.019$, and 4 (1–5) versus 1 (0–3) for mRS, $p = 0.027$, respectively), despite similar clinical backgrounds. These findings indicate that the management of NOAC treatment may be associated with not only the incidence of stroke but stroke severity and functional outcome in NOAC-associated CCE.

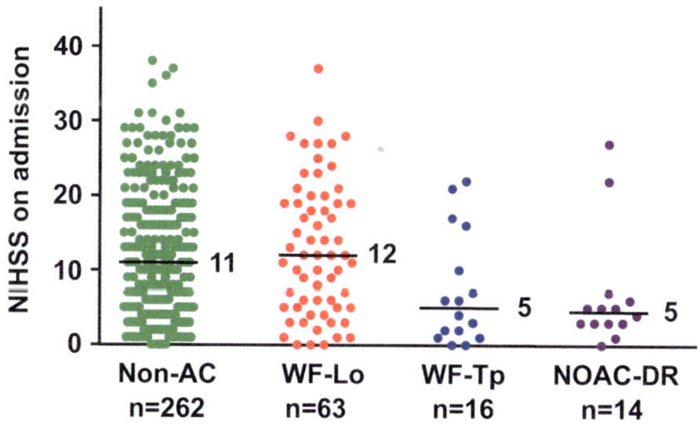

Fig. 4.3 Comparison of the National Institutes of Health Stroke Scale (NIHSS) score on admission
The NIHSS scores on non-AC (no anticoagulants), WF-Lo (warfarin treatment at lower range), WF-Tp (warfarin treatment at therapeutic range), and NOAC (NOAC treatment) groups are shown. It ranges from 0 to 42, with higher score indicating more severe stroke. The black line and number indicate median value of each group. $p = 0.006$ by the Kruskal-Wallis test. Copyright permission was obtained from the publisher of the article [30]

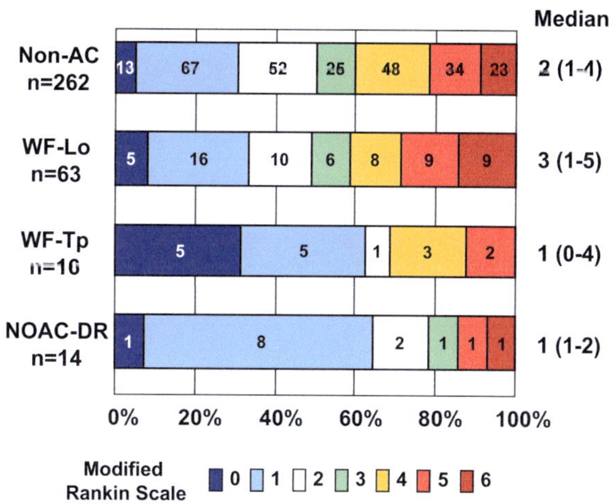

Fig. 4.4 Comparison of the modified Rankin Scale (mRS) at discharge
The mRS on non-AC (no anticoagulants), WF-Lo (warfarin treatment at lower range), WF-Tp (warfarin treatment at therapeutic range), and NOAC (NOAC treatment) groups are shown. It consists of six grades from 0 (no symptoms) to 5 (severe disability), and 6 indicates death. Median value and 25th–75th percentiles are shown in each group. Numbers in the graphs indicate the number of the patients. $p = 0.02$ by the Kruskal-Wallis test. Copyright permission was obtained from the publisher of the article [30]

References

1. Connolly SJ, Ezekowitz MD, Yusuf S, Eikelboom J, Oldgren J, Parekh A, et al. Dabigatran versus warfarin in patients with atrial fibrillation. N Engl J Med. 2009;361:1139–51.
2. Patel MR, Mahaffey KW, Garg J, Pan G, Singer DE, Hacke W, et al. Rivaroxaban versus warfarin in nonvalvular atrial fibrillation. N Engl J Med. 2011;365:883–91.
3. Granger CB, Alexander JH, McMurray JJ, Lopes RD, Hylek EM, Hanna M, et al. Apixaban versus warfarin in patients with atrial fibrillation. N Engl J Med. 2011;365:981–92.
4. Giugliano RP, Ruff CT, Braunwald E, Murphy SA, Wiviott SD, Halperin JL, et al. Edoxaban versus warfarin in patients with atrial fibrillation. N Engl J Med. 2013;369:2093–104.
5. Ruff CT, Giugliano RP, Braunwald E, Hoffman EB, Deenadayalu N, Ezekowitz MD, et al. Comparison of the efficacy and safety of new oral anticoagulants with warfarin in patients with atrial fibrillation: a meta-analysis of randomised trials. Lancet. 2014;383:955–62.
6. Yasaka M, Minematsu K, Naritomi H, Sakata T, Yamaguchi T. Predisposing factors for enlargement of intracerebral hemorrhage in patients treated with warfarin. Thromb Haemost. 2003;89:278–83.
7. Okumura K, Hagii J, Metoki N, Saito S, Shiroto H, Yasujima M, et al. Prothrombin time on admission in patients with cardioembolic stroke and intracranial hemorrhage occurring during warfarin treatment in the direct oral anticoagulant era. Rinsho Shinkeigaku = Clin Neurol. 2016;56:309–17.
8. Hagii J, Tomita H, Metoki N, Saito S, Shiroto H, Hitomi H, et al. Characteristics of intracerebral hemorrhage during rivaroxaban treatment: comparison with those during warfarin. Stroke. 2014;45:2805–7.
9. Komori M, Yasaka M, Kokuba K, Matsuoka H, Fujimoto S, Yoshida M, et al. Intracranial hemorrhage during dabigatran treatment. Circ J. 2014;78:1335–41.
10. Saji N, Kimura K, Aoki J, Uemura J, Sakamoto Y. Intracranial hemorrhage caused by non-vitamin K antagonist oral anticoagulants (NOACs)- multicenter retrospective cohort study in Japan. Circ J. 2015;79:1018–23.
11. Akiyama H, Uchino K, Hasegawa Y. Characteristics of symptomatic intracranial hemorrhage in patients receiving non-vitamin K antagonist oral anticoagulant therapy. PLoS One. 2015;10:e0132900. doi:10.1371/journal.pone.0132900.
12. Wilson D, Charidimou A, Shakeshaft C, Ambler G, White M, Cohen H, et al. Volume and functional outcome of intracerebral hemorrhage according to oral anticoagulant type. Neurology. 2016;86:360–6.
13. Hylek EM, Held C, Alexander JH, Lopes RD, De Caterina R, Wojdyla DM, et al. Major bleeding in patients with atrial fibrillation receiving apixaban or warfarin: The ARISTOTLE trial (Apixaban for Reduction in Stroke and Other Thromboembolic Events in Atrial Fibrillation): predictors, characteristics, and clinical outcomes. J Am Coll Cardiol. 2014;63:2141–7.
14. Majeed A, Hwang HG, Connolly SJ, Eikelboom JW, Ezekowitz MD, Wallentin L, et al. Management and outcomes of major bleeding during treatment with dabigatran or warfarin. Circulation. 2013;128:2325–32.
15. Purrucker JC, Capper D, Behrens L, Veltkamp R. Secondary hematoma expansion in intracerebral hemorrhage during rivaroxaban therapy. Am J Emerg Med. 2014;32:947 e3–5.
16. Simonsen CZ, Steiner T, Tietze A, Damgaard D. Dabigatran-related intracerebral hemorrhage resulting in hematoma expansion. J Stroke Cerebrovasc Dis. 2014;23:e133–4.
17. Beynon C, Sakowitz OW, Storzinger D, Orakcioglu B, Radbruch A, Potzy A, et al. Intracranial haemorrhage in patients treated with direct oral anticoagulants. Thromb Res. 2015;136:560–5.
18. Purrucker JC, Haas K, Rizos T, Khan S, Wolf M, Hennerici MG, et al. Early clinical and radiological course, management, and outcome of intracerebral hemorrhage related to new oral anticoagulants. JAMA Neurol. 2016;73:169–77.
19. Hankey GJ, Stevens SR, Piccini JP, Lokhnygina Y, Mahaffey KW, Halperin JL, et al. Intracranial hemorrhage among patients with atrial fibrillation anticoagulated with warfarin or

rivaroxaban: the rivaroxaban once daily, oral, direct factor Xa inhibition compared with vitamin K antagonism for prevention of stroke and embolism trial in atrial fibrillation. Stroke. 2014;45:1304–12.
20. Bokura H, Saika R, Yamaguchi T, Nagai A, Oguro H, Kobayashi S, et al. Microbleeds are associated with subsequent hemorrhagic and ischemic stroke in healthy elderly individuals. Stroke. 2011;42:1867–71.
21. Lovelock CE, Cordonnier C, Naka H, Al-Shahi Salman R, Sudlow CL, Sorimachi T, et al. Antithrombotic drug use, cerebral microbleeds, and intracerebral hemorrhage: a systematic review of published and unpublished studies. Stroke. 2010;41:1222–8.
22. Lee SH, Kim BJ, Roh JK. Silent microbleeds are associated with volume of primary intracerebral hemorrhage. Neurology. 2006;66:430–2.
23. Takizawa S, Tanaka F, Nishiyama K, Hasegawa Y, Nagata E, Mizuma A, et al. Protocol for cerebral microbleeds during the non-vitamin K antagonist oral anticoagulants or warfarin therapy in stroke patients with nonvalvular atrial fibrillation (CMB-NOW) study: multisite pilot trial. J Stroke Cerebrovasc Dis. 2015;24:2143–8.
24. Wilson D, Jager HR, Werring DJ. Anticoagulation for atrial fibrillation in patients with cerebral microbleeds. Curr Atheroscler Rep. 2015;17:47.
25. Hirsh J, Fuster V, Ansell J, Halperin JL. American Heart Association/American College of Cardiology Foundation guide to warfarin therapy. Circulation. 2003;107:1692–711.
26. Nozawa T, Inoue H, Iwasa A, Okumura K, Jong-dae L, Shimizu A, et al. Effects of anticoagulation intensity on hemostatic markers in patients with non-valvular atrial fibrillation. Circ J. 2004;68:29–34.
27. Hylek EM, Go AS, Chang Y, Jensvold NG, Henault LE, Selby JV, et al. Effect of intensity of oral anticoagulation on stroke severity and mortality in atrial fibrillation. N Engl J Med. 2003;349:1019–26.
28. Akao M, Chun YH, Esato M, Abe M, Tsuji H, Wada H, et al. Inappropriate use of oral anticoagulants for patients with atrial fibrillation. Circ J. 2014;78:2166–72.
29. Nakamura A, Ago T, Kamouchi M, Hata J, Matsuo R, Kuroda J, et al. Intensity of anticoagulation and clinical outcomes in acute cardioembolic stroke: the Fukuoka Stroke Registry. Stroke. 2013;44:3239–42.
30. Tomita H, Hagii J, Metoki N, Saito S, Shiroto H, Hitomi H, et al. Severity and functional outcome of patients with cardioembolic stroke occurring during non-vitamin K antagonist oral anticoagulant treatment. J Stroke Cerebrovasc Dis. 2015;24:1430–7.
31. Varin R, Mirshahi S, Mirshahi P, Klein C, Jamshedov J, Chidiac J, et al. Whole blood clots are more resistant to lysis than plasma clots--greater efficacy of rivaroxaban. Thromb Res. 2013;131:e100–9.
32. Shore S, Carey EP, Turakhia MP, Jackevicius CA, Cunningham F, Pilote L, et al. Adherence to dabigatran therapy and longitudinal patient outcomes: insights from the veterans health administration. Am Heart J. 2014;167:810–7.
33. Hayashi T, Kato Y, Fukuoka T, Deguchi I, Maruyama H, Horiuchi Y, et al. Clinical features of ischemic stroke during treatment with dabigatran: an association between decreased severity and a favorable prognosis. Intern Med. 2015;54:2433–7.

Chapter 5
Causes and Outcome in Patients with Cerebral Hemorrhage Using Antithrombotic Drugs

Michiya Kubo

Abstract Oral anticoagulants and antiplatelet drugs are increasingly being used for the prevention and treatment of thromboembolic events, especially in aging countries with aging population. We retrospectively analyzed 894 consecutive cases of intracerebral hemorrhage (ICH) treated between January 2009 and March 2015 at our stroke center, particularly focusing on comparing the use and nonuse of oral antithrombotic drugs (ATDs). Of the patients, 198 (22.2 %) received oral ATDs. Compared with only 3.2 % of the patients who did not receive ATDs, 18.7 % of those who received ATDs had worsened ICH even under intensive blood pressure-lowering management (target systolic blood pressure <140 mmHg). Poor clinical outcomes (modified Rankin scale score [mRS], 4–6) were found in 18.7 % with ATD vs. 3.2 % without ATD. Regarding clinical outcomes, poor outcomes (modified Rankin scale score [mRS], 4–6) were found in 70.8 % and 54.3 % of patients who received and those who did not receive ATDs, respectively. Much stricter control of blood pressure (<130/80 mmHg) is required to prevent ICH in patients receiving ATDs for patients with ATD in their daily lives. In order to prevent inappropriate medication of ATD and to strictly manage blood pressure, a supporting system by the regional medical network is required.

Keywords Intracerebral hemorrhage • Antithrombotic drug • Blood pressure • Clinical outcome • Regional medical network

5.1 Introduction

The incidence of intracerebral hemorrhage (ICH) is known to be higher in the East Asian countries including Japan than in the United States and European countries [1–2]. ICH is the second leading subtype of stroke after cerebral infarction. The age-standardized frequency of ICH in Japan has decreased in the past several decades (especially from 1965 to 2005), as well as that of all stroke, owing to the

M. Kubo (✉)
Department of Neurosurgery, Stroke Center, Saiseikai Toyama Hospital,
33-1 Kusunoki, Toyama-shi, Toyama 931-8533, Japan
e-mail: michiya908@gmail.com

M. Uno, K. Ogasawara (eds.), *Treatment of Non-vitamin K Antagonist Oral Anticoagulants*, DOI 10.1007/978-981-10-1878-7_5

development of excellent antihypertensive drugs [3] and a public leading prevalence of restriction of salt intake [4]. Nevertheless, in the last decade, the incidence of ICH has been stable not only in Japan but also worldwide, and ICH has become the leading cause of disability [5–7]. In recent years, this is explained as follows: the decrease in the incidence of ICH due to hypertension has been offset by the increase in the incidence of ICH related to oral antithrombotic drug use [8–10].

This chapter provides community-based data on ICH in the Toyama area (mid-north area in Japan) and the relationship between ICH and oral antithrombotic drug use.

5.2 Analysis of the Incidence of ICH in the Toyama Area, Japan

5.2.1 Background and Management of ICH

This study was conducted at the stroke center of Saiseikai Toyama Hospital, Toyama, Japan, to which 55–60 % of patients with acute stroke in the area were transported by ambulance (600–700 cases per year). Toyama has a population of more than 500,000 and is a typical aging society in Japan, where the population of residents older than 65 years is 29.7 % [4]. The average daily salt intake among residents is 11.3 g for men and 9.7 g for women [4].

The basic diagnostic principle for ICH is to perform computed tomography (CT) initially, followed by another CT imaging after 3 h. Management of ICH among the patients includes the following: (1) strict blood pressure-lowering control (systolic blood pressure ≤ 140 mmHg) with intravenous administration of nitroglycerin and diltiazem hydrochloride; (2) intravenous administration of antifibrinolytic agents, including carbazochrome sodium sulfonate hydrate and tranexamic acid; and (3) intravenous injection of vitamin K to counteract the anticoagulant effect of anticoagulation therapy, mainly at the emergency department and/or the stroke care unit.

The study duration was 6 years and 3 months (January 2009–March 2015).

5.2.2 Data Source and Searches

In this period, consecutive 892 patients with nontraumatic ICH (510 men, 57.2 %; 382 women, 42.8 %; age range 21–100 years old [mean, 70.8 years]) were evaluated based on medical records, radiological images, data from the hospital stroke database, use of oral antithrombotic drug (dose and type/name), location of the ICH, enlargement of hematoma after hospitalization, risk factors, outcome on discharge (modified Rankin scale), and reasons for undergoing antithrombotic therapy.

Patients with ICH due to arteriovenous malformation or cerebral aneurysm were excluded.

In this study period, ischemic stroke accounts for 68.1 %; ICH, for 24.7 %; and subarachnoid hemorrhage, for 7.2 % of the subjects. The incidence of ICH was markedly higher in the United States and European countries (10–15 %) [7] but was nearly average in East Asia.

5.2.3 ICH with Oral Anticoagulation and/or Antiplatelet Therapy

In our series, 198 patients (22.2 %) with ICH taking antithrombotic therapy were identified (Fig. 5.1). Recently, the use of antithrombotic (anticoagulant and/or antiplatelet) drugs has been considered a risk factor of ICH [8–10]. The incidence of intracranial hemorrhage during antithrombotic therapy has increased from 15.2 % to 18.5 % in the recent 6 years in Japan [5, 11, 13]. It has been reported to reach even 27.0 % by another multicenter study in Japan [12].

Regarding the types of antithrombotic drugs in our series, ICH that occurred under antiplatelet, anticoagulation, and combined antiplatelet and anticoagulation therapies accounted for 69.2 % (137/198), 18.7 % (37 /198), and 12.1 % (24/198) of the treated cases, respectively.

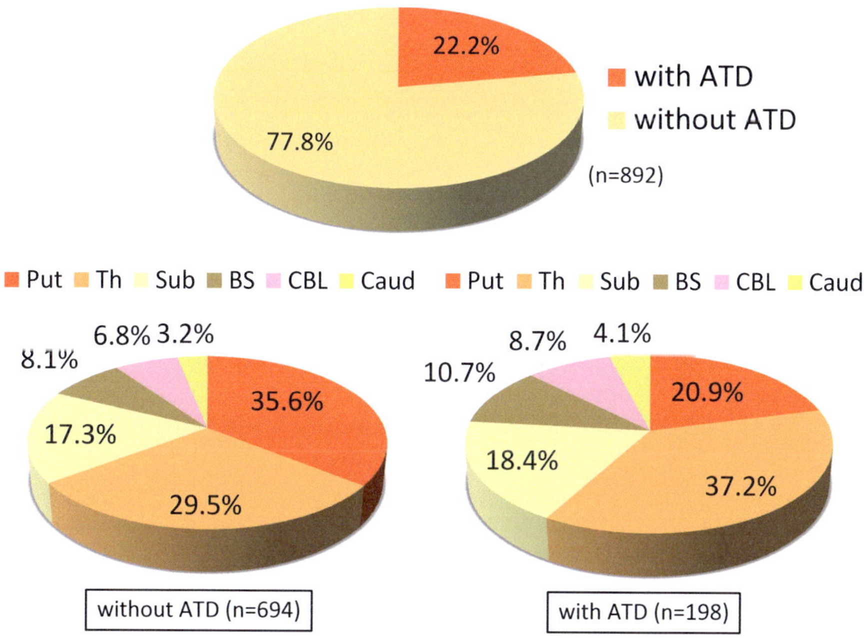

Fig. 5.1 [*upper*] Intracerebral hemorrhage with/without ATD (ATD: antithrombotic drugs). [*lower*] Distribution of locations of ICH without (*left*) and with (*right*) ATD

Among the 137 ICH cases that occurred under antiplatelet therapy, 117 (85.4 %) were under monotherapy (aspirin, 78.6 %; clopidogrel, 6.8 %; cilostazol, 6.0 %; others, 9.4 %), and 20 (14.6 %) were under dual antiplatelet therapy (DAPT).

Among the 37 ICH cases that occurred under anticoagulation therapy, 33 (89.2 %) were under warfarin and four (10.8 %) were under non-vitamin K antagonist oral anticoagulants (NOACs), which included three cases under rivaroxaban and one under apixaban.

In Japan, four types of NOAC are currently available. Dabigatran was approved in 2011; rivaroxaban, in 2012; apixaban, in 2013; and edoxaban, in December 2014. Hence it is inadequate to compare the incidence of ICH treated with anticoagulation therapy among four different types of NOAC.

5.2.4 The Location of the ICH Cases that Occurred Under Antithrombotic Therapy

The predominant location of ICH is known to vary with age and population.

In the United States, Europe, and Australia, deep cerebral ICH (putamen, thalamus, and caudate nucleus) is the most common (36–49 %), but is closely followed by lobar hemorrhage (34–52 %). In Japan, lobar hemorrhage accounts for 15 %, and deep ICH accounts for 69 % of cases [1, 18–20]. Among the deep cerebral ICH cases, putaminal hemorrhage was predominant in persons younger than 50 years (putamen, 41.9 %; thalamus, 11.7 %). However, of those older than 50 years, 27.2 % had thalamic hemorrhage (putamen 28.2 %) [5].

Our study demonstrates the distribution of the locations of ICH as follows (Fig. 5.1): (patients with antithrombotic therapy, n = 198) 37.2 % in the thalamus, 20.9 % in the putamen, 18.4 % in the subcortex (lobar type), 10.7 % in the brainstem, 8.7 % in the cerebellum, 4.1 % in the caudate nucleus, and others and (patients without antithrombotic therapy, n = 694) 29.5 % in the thalamus, 35.6 % in the putamen, 17.3 % in the subcortex (lobar type), 8.1 % in the brainstem, 6.8 % in the cerebellum, 3.2 % in the caudate nucleus, and others. A higher incidence rate of thalamic hemorrhage under antithrombotic therapy means a higher incidence rate of elderly patients in the group [5].

The types of antithrombotic drugs and location of ICH in our series are as follows: (patients with antiplatelet drug only, n = 137) 40.1 % in the thalamus, 19.0 % in the subcortex (lobar type), 18.2 % in the putamen, 10.2 % in the brainstem, 8.8 % in the cerebellum, 3.6 % in the caudate nucleus, and others and (patients with anticoagulant or both, n = 59) 30.5 % in the thalamus, 27.1 % in the putamen, 16.9% in the subcortex (lobar type), 11.9 % in the brainstem, 8.5 % in the cerebellum, 5.1 % in the caudate nucleus, and others.

5.2.5 Clinical Outcomes

ICH is sometimes clinically devastating. Mortality has been reported to range from 40 to 50 % in any study [1–14]. In our study, the mortality rates were 25.8 % and 15.4 % in the patients who were receiving and those who were not receiving antithrombotic therapy in spite of strict management of blood pressure and hemostasis. In the patients who were receiving and those not receiving antithrombotic therapy, poor outcomes (modified Rankin scale score, 4–6) at discharge were observed in 70.8 % and 54.3 %, respectively, and very poor outcomes (modified Rankin scale score, 5 or 6) were observed in 45.5 % and 28.5 %, respectively (Fig. 5.2).

5.2.6 Reasons for Taking Antiplatelet and/or Anticoagulation Drugs

Among the 198 patients with ICH who were receiving antithrombotic therapy, 57 (28.8 %) were taking antithrombotic drugs for prevention of recurrence of cerebral ischemia. Another 57 patients (28.8 %) had atrial fibrillation (AF) for stroke prevention, but nine of them were receiving antiplatelet therapy in spite of the required anticoagulation therapy (Fig. 5.2). Forty patients (20.2 %) were taking

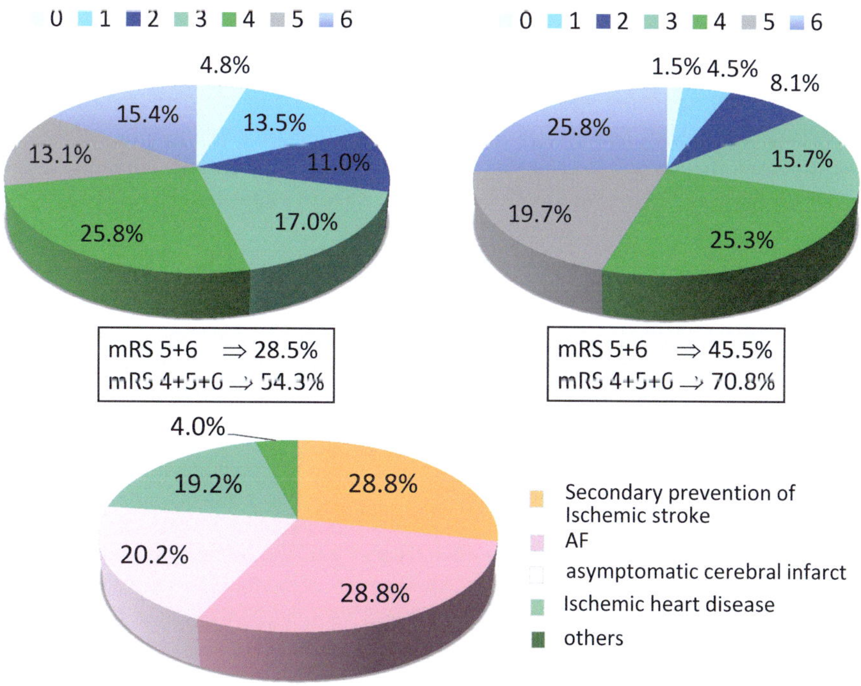

Fig. 5.2 [upper] Clinical outcome of ICH without (*left*) and with (*right*) ATD. [*lower*] Reasons of taking ATD

antithrombotic drugs under the diagnosis of asymptomatic cerebral infarction on a radiological image only or because of a risk factor of ischemic stroke (diabetes mellitus, hyperlipidemia, and hypertension). Thirty-eight patients (19.2 %) were treated for ischemic heart disease (mainly after coronary stenting). The remaining eight patients (4.0 %) received treatments of peripheral arterial disease (mainly the lower extremities), deep venous thrombosis, and retinal arterial occlusion.

In order to prevent inappropriate medication with antithrombotic drugs and to strictly manage their blood pressures within lower levels [16], a supporting system by the regional medical network is required. Based on these results, an awareness campaign is required for home physicians not to prescribe antithrombotic drugs for asymptomatic cerebral infarction, to treat with appropriate doses of anticoagulants not antiplatelet drugs, strict blood pressure control within lower levels for patients with antithrombotic therapy [16].

5.3 Enlargement of Hematoma and Antithrombotic Therapy

5.3.1 *Incidence of Expansion of Hematoma After Admission*

Enlargement of ICH on follow-up CT at or within 3 h after admission was observed in 59 cases (6.6 %) in our study (Fig. 5.3).

Compared with the non-antithrombotic drug users (3.2 %, 22/694), the antithrombotic drug users (18.7 %, 37/198) had a significantly higher incidence rate of enlargement of ICH ($p < 0.01$) in our series (Fig. 5.3).

Hematoma expansion was found in 12.4 % (17/137) of the patients who were receiving antiplatelet therapy, 32.4 % (12/37) of those receiving anticoagulation therapy, and 36.4 % (8/22) of those receiving combined antiplatelet and anticoagulation therapy (Fig. 5.4). We identified only one case of expansion of ICH (thalamic hemorrhage) under NOAC therapy (rivaroxaban), in which the size of the hematoma was small (<10 mL) and the growth of ICH was unremarkable (Fig. 5.5). The reported clinical characteristics of ICH under NOAC therapy were smaller and rarer expansion than those under warfarin therapy [15].

5.3.2 *Growth of Hematoma Under Antithrombotic Therapy and Location of ICH*

Recent reports divided the locations of ICH just into the lobar type and the deep types [17–20]. However, in this study, the growth of hematoma was observed in 19.2 % (14/73) of the cases in the thalamus and 53.7 % (22/41) of the cases in the

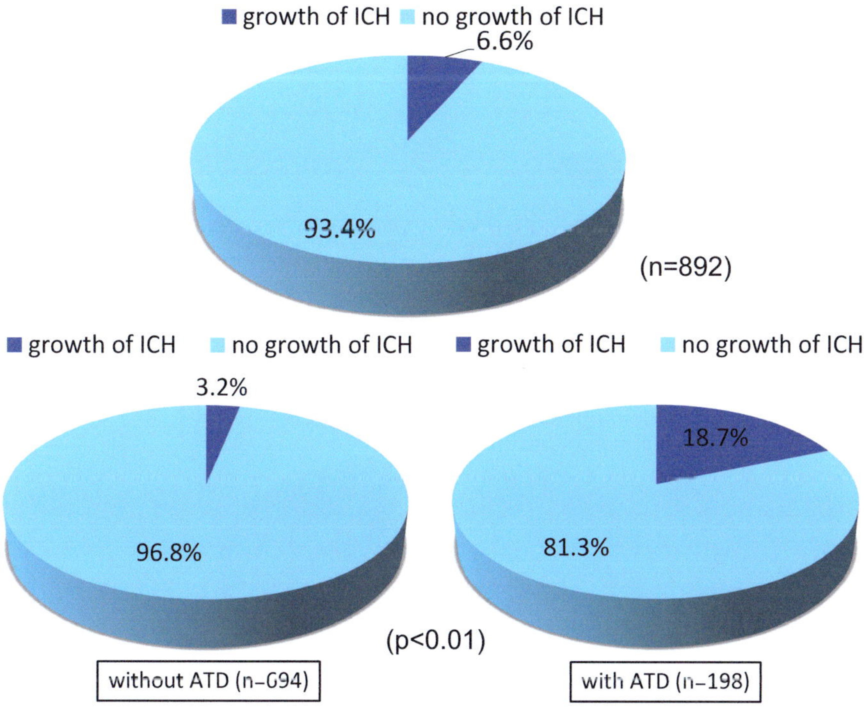

Fig. 5.3 [*upper*] Growth of ICH on follow-up CT 3 h after admission. [*lower*] Growth of ICH without (*left*) and with (*right*) ATD

putamen (Fig. 5.6), even if they were contained in the same deep areas ($p < 0.01$). A higher incidence of putaminal hemorrhage may result from the distribution of tissue factor (TF) in the brain because TF is numerously expressed in the brain, especially in the glial cells [22].

Expansion of hemorrhage was observed in the other locations, including 27.8 % (10/36) in the subcortex (lobar hemorrhage), 33.3 % (7/21) in the brainstem, 29.4 % (5/17) in the cerebellum, and 19.2 % (1/8) in the caudate nucleus.

5.4 Antithrombotic Therapy: Balance of Benefit and ICH Risk

The prevalence of AF is a highly age-associated risk factor of ischemic stroke [21]. Oral anticoagulant therapy for AF can largely reverse the risk of ischemic stroke. However, the incidence of oral anticoagulant-associated ICH is likely to increase.

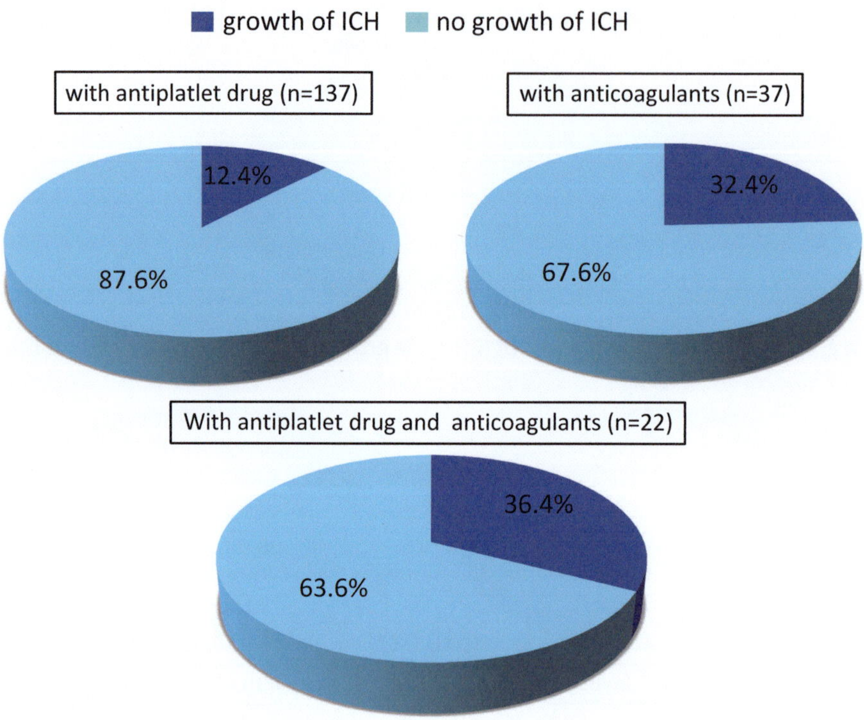

Fig. 5.4 Growth of ICH with antiplatelet drugs [*upper left*], anticoagulants [*upper right*], antiplatelet drugs and anticoagulants [*lower*]

ICH is caused by multiple factors, but hypertension remains the most important risk factor. Hypertension (including untreated hypertension) was identified in 89.7 % of the patients in our study. Western countries have higher incidence rates of lobar hemorrhage, followed by cerebral amyloid angiopathy, particularly among elderly patients. The use of antithrombotic drugs, mainly warfarin and antiplatelets, has recently emerged as a newly focused risk factor of ICH. Data on the use of NOAC for ICH are scarce, although several characteristics of ICH cases that occurred under NOAC therapy have been identified, including less frequent (0.23–0.49 %), smaller in size, and rarely enlarged as compared with those under warfarin therapy (0.74–0.85 %) [23–26].

To prevent ICH in patients receiving antithrombotic drugs, several aspects require attention during medication as follows: appropriate selection of antithrombotic drugs, adequate blood pressure control [16], and appropriate indication for antithrombotic therapy.

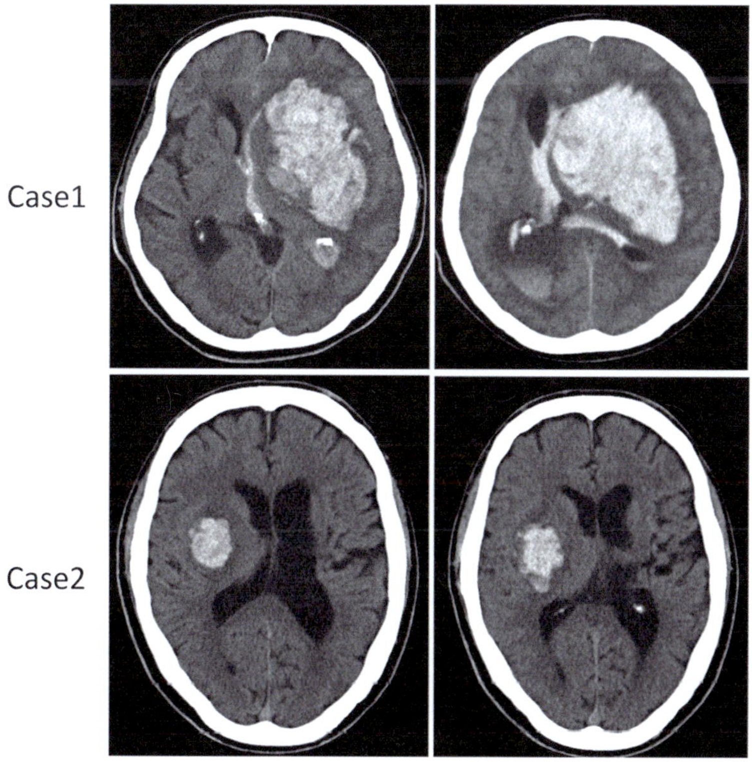

Fig. 5.5 Characteristics of ICH on CT: [*upper*] Case1. Left putaminal hemorrhage with warfarin on admission (*left*) and follow-up (*right*). [*lower*] Case2. Right thalamic hemorrhage with NOAC (rivaroxaban) on admission (*left*) and follow-up (*right*)

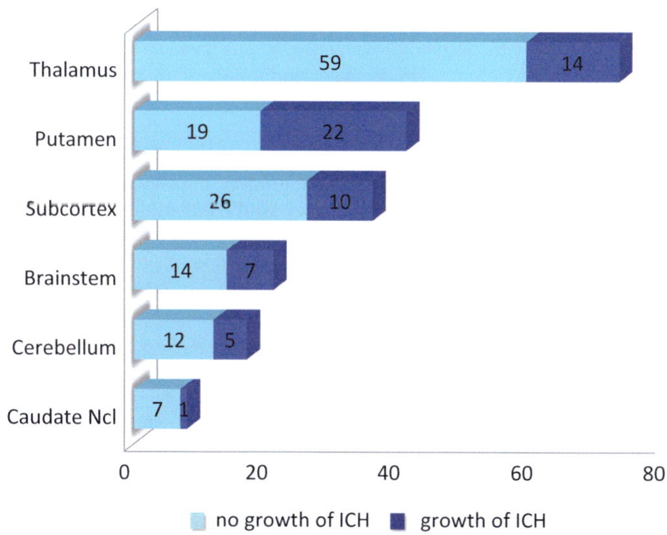

Fig. 5.6 The rate of growth of hematoma at each location of ICH

Acknowledgments The author appreciates the staff, Horie Y, Okamoto S, Hori E, Umemura K, Shibata T, and Hori S, in Stroke Center, Saiseikai Toyama Hospital, and Kuroda S and Kuwayama N, the Department of Neurosurgery, University of Toyama, for their support of this study.

References

1. Inagawa T, Ohbayashi N, Takechi A, Shibukawa M, Yahara K. Primary intracerebral hemorrhage in Izumo City, Japan: incidence rates and outcome in relation to the site of hemorrhage. Neurosurgery. 2003;53:1283–98.
2. Jiang B, Wang W, Chen H, et al. Incidence and trends of stroke and its subtypes in China: results from hree large cities. Stroke. 2006;37:63–5.
3. PROGRESS Collaborative Group. Randomised trial of perindopril-based blood-pressure-lowering regimen among 6105 individuals with previous stroke or transient ischemic attack. Lancet. 2001;358:1033–41.
4. Ministry of Health, Labour and Welfare: The Japanese National vital statistics 1996–2015.
5. Takizawa S. Incidence of intracerebral hemorrhage: Causes, location, age, and sex. Kobayashi S, editor. Stroke Data Base 2015. Nakayama-shoten, 2015, p.132-133.
6. Ikram MA, Wieberdink RG, Koudstaal PJ. International epidemiology of intracerebral hemorrhage. Current Atherosclerosis Report. 2012;14:303–6.
7. Feigin VL, Lawes CM, Bennett DA, Barker-Collo SL, Parag V. Worldwide stroke incidence and early case fatality reported in 56 population-based studies: a systematic review. Lancet Neurol. 2009;8:355–69.
8. Yasaka M, Okada Y. Management of intracranial hemorrhage during anticoagulant therapy with warfarin or novel anticoagulants. Clin Neurol. 2012;52:1113–6.
9. Hart RG, Tonarelli SB, Pearce LA. Avoiding central nervous system bleeding during antithrombotic therapy: recent data and ideas. Stroke. 2005;36:1588–93.
10. Toyoda K, Yasaka M, Uchiyama S, Bleeding with Antithrombotic Therapy (BAT) Study Group, et al. Blood pressure levels and bleeding events during antithrombotic therapy : the Bleeding with Antithrombotic Therapy (BAT) Study. Stroke. 2010;41:1440–4.
11. Suzuki R, Toyoda K, Minematsu K. Antithrombotic therapy and intracerebral hemorrhage: clinical outcome, location, enlargement of hematoma, and clinical outcome. Kobayashi S, editor. Stroke Data Base 2015. Nakayama-shoten, 2015, pp.144-5.
12. Toyoda K, Yasaka M, Iwade K, Nagata K, Koretsune Y, Sakamoto T, et al. Bleeding with Antithrombotic Therapy (BAT) Study Group: dual antithrombotic therapy increases severe bleeding events in patients with stroke and cardiovascular disease: a prospective, multicenter, observational study. Stroke. 2008;39:1740–5.
13. Toyoda K, Yasaka M, Nagata K, Nagao T, Gotoh J, Sakamoto T, Bleeding with Antithrombotic Therapy Study Group, et al. Antithrombotic therapy influences location, enlargement, and mortality from intracerebral hemorrhage: the Bleeding with Antithrombotic Therapy (BAT) Retrospective Study. Cerebrovasc Dis. 2009;27:151–9.
14. Tanaka H, Ueda Y, Date C, Baba T, Yamashita H, Hayashi M, et al. Incidence of stroke in Shibata, Japan: 1976–1978. Stroke. 1981;12:460–6.
15. Akiyama H, Uchino K, Hasegawa Y. Characteristics of symptomatic intracranial hemorrhage in patients receiving non-vitamin K antagonist oral anticoagulant therapy; 2015. doi:http://dx.doi.org/10.1371/journal.pone.0132900.
16. Toyoda K, Yasaka M, Uchiyama S, Nagao T, Goto J, Nagata K, et al. Blood pressure levels and bleeding events during antithrombotic therapy: the Bleeding with Antithrombotic Therapy (BAT) Study. Stroke. 2010;41:1440–4.
17. Cucchiara B, Messe S, Sansing L, Kasner S, Lyden P, Investigators CHANT. Hematoma growth in oral anticoagulant related intracerebral hemorrhage. Stroke. 2008;39:2993–6.

18. Flaherty ML, Woo D, Haverbusch M, et al. Racial variations in location and risk of intracerebral hemorrhage. Stroke. 2005;36:934–7.
19. Fogelholm R, Nuutila M, Vuorela A-L. Primary intracerebral haemorrhage in the Jyvaskyla region, central Finland, 1985–89: incidence, case fatality rate, and functional outcome. J Neurol Neurosurg Psychiatry. 1992;55:546–52.
20. Nilsson O, Lindgren A, Stahl N, Brandt L, Saveland H. Incidence of intracerebral and subarachnoid haemorrhage in southern Sweden. J Neurol Neurosurg Psychiatry. 2000;69:601–7.
21. Inoue H, Fujiki A, Origasa H, Ogawa S, Okumura K, Kubota I, et al. Prevalence of atrial fibrillation in the general population of Japan: an analysis based on periodic health examination. Int J Cardiol. 2009;137:102–7.
22. Drake TA, Morrissey GH, Edgington TS. Selective cellular expression of tissue factor in human tissues. Implications for disorders of hemostasis and thrombosis. Am J Pathol. 1989;134:1087–97.
23. Connolly SJ, Ezekowitz MD, Yusef F, Eikelboom J, Oldgren J, Parekh A, et al. Dabigatran versus warfarin in patients with atrial fibrillation. N Eng J Med. 2008;361:1740–5.
24. Patel MR, Mahaffey KW, Garg J, Pan G, Singer DE, Hacke W, et al. Rivaroxaban versus warfarin in nonvalvular atrial fibrillation. N Eng J Med. 2011;365:883–91.
25. Granger CB, Alexander JH, McMurray JJ, Lopes RD, Hylek EM, Hanna M, et al. Apixaban versus warfarin in patients with atrial fibrillation. N Eng J Med. 2011;365:981–92.
26. Giugliano RP, Ruff CT, Braunwald E, Murphy SA, Wiviott SD, Halperin JL, et al. Edoxaban versus warfarin in patients with atrial fibrillation. N Eng J Med. 2013;369:2093–104.

Chapter 6
Secondary Prevention of Cerebral Infarct

Verification of Appropriateness in Choices of Anticoagulant by Comparison of Current and Previous Treatment Results

Akira Nakamizo, Shinya Yamaguchi, Masato Osaki, and Shigeru Fujimoto

Abstract We hypothesized that the treatment results for secondary prevention of cerebral infarct in patients with AF have improved as the therapeutic availability of anticoagulants has expanded, if the choice of drug and selection of dose were appropriate for the individual. To test this hypothesis, we analyzed a total of 425 patients who had been admitted due to stroke or TIA and had been prescribed anticoagulants on first discharge. Patients were divided into four groups according to the number of anticoagulants available in our hospital: warfarin alone as Period 1; warfarin and dabigatran as Period 2; warfarin, dabigatran, and rivaroxaban as Period 3; and warfarin, dabigatran, rivaroxaban, and apixaban as Period 4. We made it a principle to avoid unnecessary dose reduction as well as to choose the NOAC that did not meet the dose-reduction criteria for each individual patient in cases where we decided to treat patients with NOACs in Period 4 according to the treatment results in Periods 1–3. The incidences of recurrent stroke were 10.2 %, 12.0 %, 8.8 %, and 4.7 % in Periods 1, 2, 3, and 4, respectively. During the entire follow-up period, five cerebral infarcts occurred in patients treated with low-dose NOACs, with none in patients on standard-dose NOACs. In Period 4, no patient treated with NOACs experienced recurrent ischemic stroke. One small intracranial hemorrhage occurred in the patient treated with low-dose apixaban in Period 4. Comparisons of current and previous treatment results may be helpful to self-check the validity of the decision-making process in individual hospitals and can contribute to improved outcomes for secondary prevention of cerebral infarct.

Keywords NOAC • Non-vitamin K antagonist oral anticoagulant • Atrial fibrillation • Cerebral infarct • Secondary prevention

---

A. Nakamizo (✉) • S. Yamaguchi • M. Osaki • S. Fujimoto
Department of Neurosurgery, Stroke Center, Steel Memorial Yawata Hospital,
1-1-1 Harunomachi, Yahata higashi-ku, Kitakyushu, 805-0050, Japan
e-mail: nakamizo@ns.med.kyushu-u.ac.jp

M. Uno, K. Ogasawara (eds.), *Treatment of Non-vitamin K Antagonist Oral Anticoagulants*, DOI 10.1007/978-981-10-1878-7_6

6.1 Introduction

6.1.1 Development of NOACs

Non-vitamin K antagonist oral anticoagulants (NOACs) have become available as an alternative for warfarin in both primary and secondary prevention of cerebral infarct in non-valvular atrial fibrillation (AF); dabigatran was licensed in Japan in 2011, followed by rivaroxaban, apixaban, and edoxaban in 2012, 2013, and 2014, respectively. Based on four warfarin-based randomized controlled trials (RCTs) of NOACs versus warfarin for thromboprophylaxis in AF, the Randomized Evaluation of Long-Term Anticoagulation Therapy (RE-LY) trial, the Rivaroxaban Once-Daily Oral Direct Factor Xa Inhibition Compared with Vitamin K Antagonism for Prevention of Stroke and Embolism Trial in Atrial Fibrillation (ROCKET-AF) trial, the Apixaban for Reduction in Stroke and Other Thromboembolic Events in Atrial Fibrillation (ARISTOTLE) trial, and the Effective Anticoagulation with Factor Xa Next Generation in Atrial Fibrillation Thrombolysis in Myocardial Infarction 48 (ENGAGE AF-TIMI 48) trial, these four NOACs have been shown to be non-inferior or superior to warfarin in the prevention of stroke and systemic embolism [1–4].

A recent meta-analysis showed that NOACs significantly reduced the risk of stroke and systemic embolism by 19 % compared with warfarin (relative risk (RR) 0.81, 95 % confidence interval (CI) 0.73–0.91; $P < 0.0001$), along with intracranial hemorrhage (RR 0.48, 95 %CI 0.39–0.59; $P < 0.0001$), and all-cause mortality (RR 0.90, 95 %CI 0.85–0.95; $P = 0.0003$), but increased the risk of gastrointestinal bleeding (RR 1.25, 95 %CI 1.01–1.55; $P = 0.04$) in patients with AF [5].

6.1.2 Thromboembolic and Hemorrhagic Risks in Secondary Prevention

Both thromboembolic and hemorrhagic risks are considered to be higher with secondary prevention of cerebral infarct than with primary prevention. Some risk factors are shared between thromboembolic and hemorrhagic events. $CHADS_2$ score [6] (presence of congestive heart failure, hypertension, age ≥ 75 years, diabetes mellitus (1 point each), history of stroke or TIA (2 points)) shares the subitems of hypertension, age, and previous stroke with HAS-BLED score [7] (hypertension, abnormal renal/liver function, stroke, bleeding history or predisposition, labile INR, elderly (≥65 years old) or frail, drugs/alcohol concomitantly), which has been validated and is commonly used for prediction of the risk of hemorrhagic events [7–9]. Sub-analysis of the RE-LY trial demonstrated that stroke or systemic embolism as well as major bleeding occurred more frequently in patients with previous stroke or TIA compared to those without such a history [10].

6.1.3 Increasing Choice of Anticoagulants for Secondary Prevention

For secondary prevention, four NOACs and warfarin are all candidate anticoagulants recommended by the guidelines for pharmacotherapy for AF [11]. Subanalyses and a meta-analysis of the RE-LY, ROCKET-AF, and ARISTOTLE trials demonstrated that dabigatran, rivaroxaban, and apixaban were all non inferior to warfarin in patients with prior stroke or TIA [10, 12–14]. However, there is little evidence to suggest which NOAC is superior to the others in secondary prevention of cerebral infarcts.

The absence of head-to-head comparisons of NOACs makes it difficult to assess which NOAC might be superior to the others for individual patients [15, 16]. Several investigators have conducted indirect comparisons of the results of RCTs using network meta-analysis [17–19], but the validity of the results may be limited because of the differences in study designs and patient profiles [15]. For example, patients enrolled in ROCKET-AF had a higher risk of thromboembolic events (mean $CHADS_2$ score, 3.5; median time in therapeutic range (TTR), 58 %) than patients in RE-LY (mean $CHADS_2$ score, 2.1; median TTR, 67 %), ARISTOTLE (mean $CHADS_2$ score, 2.1; median TTR, 66 %), or ENGAGE AF-TIMI 48 (mean $CHADS_2$ score, 2.8; median TTR, 68 %) [1–4].

At present, we have to decide which drug should be used for a patient based on clinical experience and suggestions based on the results of RCTs and meta-analyses [20, 21].

6.1.4 Hypothesis: AF Patients Benefit from the Increasing Number of NOACs Available

Nevertheless, the increase in the number of anticoagulants available allows us to choose a drug that we expect to be optimal for the individual patient from among four NOACs and warfarin in consideration of patient characteristics such as age, body weight, renal function, bleeding tendency, patient characteristics, drug tolerability, cost, and likelihood to adhere to treatment.

We hypothesized that the treatment results for secondary prevention of cerebral infarct in patients with AF have improved as the therapeutic availability of anticoagulants has expanded, if the choice of drug and selection of dose were appropriate for the individual. To test this hypothesis, we analyzed the outcomes of patients with previous stroke or TIA treated using anticoagulants for the prevention of secondary stroke and verified whether the treatment results in our hospital have improved as the number of anticoagulants available has increased. In addition, we discuss factors that may influence treatment results, which can lead to better clinical outcomes for AF patients with previous stroke or TIA.

6.2 Verification of Treatment Results for Secondary Prevention

6.2.1 *Patients*

A total of 425 patients who had been admitted due to stroke or TIA and had been prescribed anticoagulants on first discharge for the secondary prevention of cerebral infarction were extracted from the database of all acute stroke patients admitted to our hospital from February 2008 to December 2014.

Patients were divided into four groups according to the number of anticoagulants available in our hospital: warfarin alone as Period 1 (February 2008 to March 2011); warfarin and dabigatran as Period 2 (April 2011 to April 2012); warfarin, dabigatran, and rivaroxaban as Period 3 (May 2012 to February 2013); and warfarin, dabigatran, rivaroxaban, and apixaban as Period 4 (March 2013 to December 2014).

Patient profiles varied among periods (Table 6.1). The risk of thromboembolic events in patients was higher in Period 3 than in the other periods. Patients with low body weight, low creatinine clearance, high modified Rankin scale (mRS) score, and high National Institutes of Health stroke scale score were more common in Period 3 than in the other periods. Patients with chronic kidney disease were more common in Periods 3 and 4 than in the other periods. $CHADS_2$ score gradually increased from Period 1 to 4.

Table 6.1 Baseline characteristics

Variables	Period 1 (n = 185)	Period 2 (n = 80)	Period 3 (n = 62)	Period 4 (n = 98)	P value
Age (yrs)	76.7	77.6	76.7	78.3	0.6806
Sex (male ratio, %)	55.7	50.0	51.6	58.2	0.6838
Body weight (kg)	55.9	55.9	52.9	55.1	0.4011
CCr (mL/min)	57.1	60.1	48.3	51.8	0.0474
mRS	2.2	2.3	2.5	2.4	0.7016
NIHSS	4.5	4.2	5.4	4.1	0.6792
Antiplatelet treatment (%)	35.1	18.8	29.0	23.5	0.0272
Smoking (%)	15.9	8.8	9.7	14.3	0.3281
Alcohol (%)	40.5	32.5	21.0	35.7	0.0364
AF (%)	64.9	68.8	74.2	67.4	0.5818
DM (%)	26.5	26.3	30.7	27.6	0.7409
HT (%)	68.1	67.5	75.8	79.6	0.1346
CKD (%)	2.7	5.0	9.7	7.1	0.1397
DL (%)	34.6	27.5	35.5	41.8	0.2575
$CHADS_2$ score	3.81	3.85	3.89	3.92	0.8096

CCr creatinine clearance, *mRS* modified Rankin scale, *NIHSS* NIH stroke scale, *AF* atrial fibrillation, *DM* diabetes mellitus, *HT* hypertension, *CKD* chronic kidney disease, *DL* dyslipidemia

Table 6.2 Mean $CHADS_2$ score and anticoagulants

	W	$D_{110mgBID}$	$D_{150mgBID}$	R_{10mgOD}	R_{15mgOD}	$A_{2.5mgBID}$	A_{5mgBID}	P value
Period 1	3.81 (n = 185)							N/A
Period 2	3.81 (n = 57)	4.10 (n = 20)	3.00 (n = 3)					0.1378
Period 3	4.00 (n = 48)	3.80 (n = 5)	3.00 (n = 1)	3.67 (n = 3)	3.20 (n = 5)			0.3363
Period 4	3.95 (n = 64)	4.25 (n = 4)	2.00 (n = 1)	3.00 (n = 1)	3.38 (n = 8)	4.44 (n = 9)	3.82 (n = 11)	0.0872

W warfarin, *D* dabigatran, *R* rivaroxaban, *A* apixaban

6.2.2 *Choice of Drug and Dose Selection for NOACs*

Premised on strict adherence to indications and dose regulatory recommendations for each NOAC to avoid adverse effects such as major bleeding, intracranial hemorrhage, and gastrointestinal bleeding, we made it a principle to avoid unnecessary dose reduction as well as to choose the NOAC that did not meet the dose-reduction criteria for each individual patient in cases where we decided to treat patients with NOACs in Period 4 according to the treatment results in Periods 1–3.

As a result, 29 %, 23 %, and 35 % of patients in Periods 2, 3, and 4, respectively, received NOACs as an alternative to warfarin. Likewise, the proportion of standard-dose to low-dose NOACs increased from Period 2 to Period 4. Thirteen percent, 43 %, and 59 % of NOACs were used at standard doses in Periods 2, 3, and 4, respectively. In Period 4, patients with high $CHADS_2$ scores tended to be allocated to receive low-dose dabigatran or low-dose apixaban, whereas other patients were aggressively allocated to receive high-dose NOACs (Table 6.2).

6.3 Treatment Results

6.3.1 *Overall Treatment Results*

The incidences of recurrent stroke, all-cause death, intracranial hemorrhage, hemorrhagic complications, and cardiovascular events within 1 year after first-time stroke in each period were analyzed. All analyses were performed according to the intention-to-treat principle. Kaplan-Meier survival analysis was used to compare the incidences.

Recurrent stroke within 1 year was significantly decreased in Period 4. The incidences of recurrent stroke were 10.2 %, 12.0 %, 8.8 %, and 4.7 % in Periods 1, 2, 3, and 4, respectively (Fig. 6.1a). Incidences of all-cause death were 11.4 %, 7.8 %, 15.0 %, and 13.2 % in Periods 1, 2, 3, and 4, respectively (Fig. 6.1b). Incidences of recurrent stroke or all-cause death were 18.4 %, 15.6 %, 23.3 %, and 15.2 % in Periods 1, 2, 3, and 4, respectively (Fig. 6.1c).

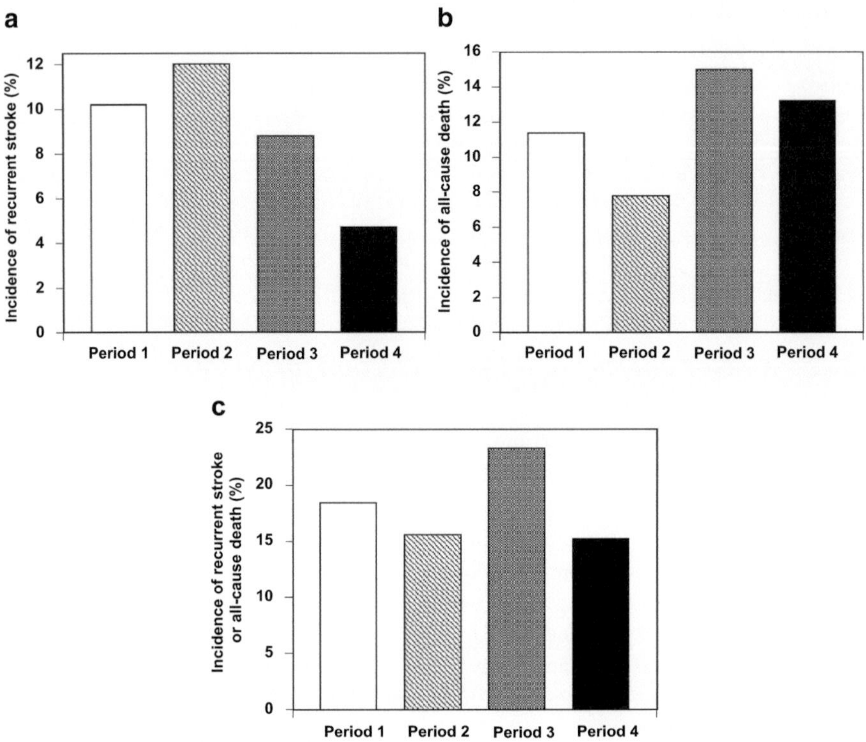

Fig. 6.1 Incidences of recurrent stroke (**a**), all-cause death (**b**), and recurrent stroke or all-cause death (**c**) within 1 year after first-time stroke in each period

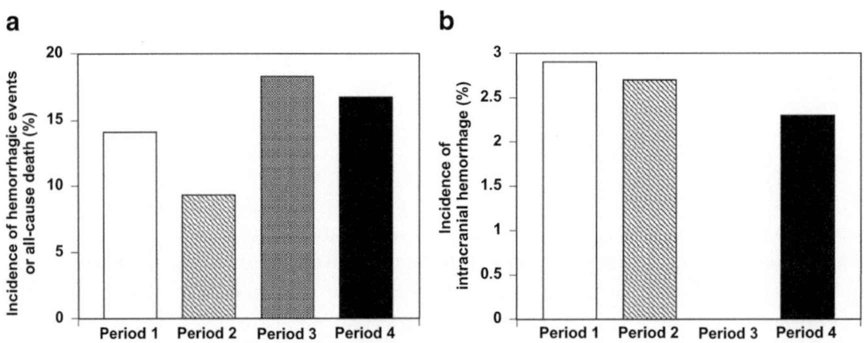

Fig. 6.2 Incidences of hemorrhagic event or all-cause death (**a**) and intracranial hemorrhage (**b**) within 1 year after first-time stroke in each period

In Periods 3 and 4, the incidence of hemorrhagic complications or all-cause death within 1 year increased slightly (Fig. 6.2a), whereas the incidence of intracranial hemorrhage decreased (Fig. 6.2b). Incidences of cardiovascular event within 1 year were 7.6 %, 17.5 %, 22.5 %, and 15.3 %, in Periods 1, 2, 3, and 4, respectively.

6.3.2 Benefit of NOACs on Disabled Patients

We tried to determine whether the benefit from the increasing number of NOACs available differs according to patient disability. Patients were divided into two groups with mRS 0–2 and mRS 3–5 at first-time discharge. Mean $CHADS_2$ score was higher in patients with mRS 3–4 than in those with mRS 0–2 (Fig. 6.3). Among patients with mRS 0–2, the incidence of recurrent stroke gradually declined from Period 1 to 4 (Fig. 6.4 and Table 6.3). On the other hand, among patients with mRS 3–5, the incidence of recurrent stroke was dramatically suppressed in Period 4 compared to in the other periods. The increasing number of anticoagulants available

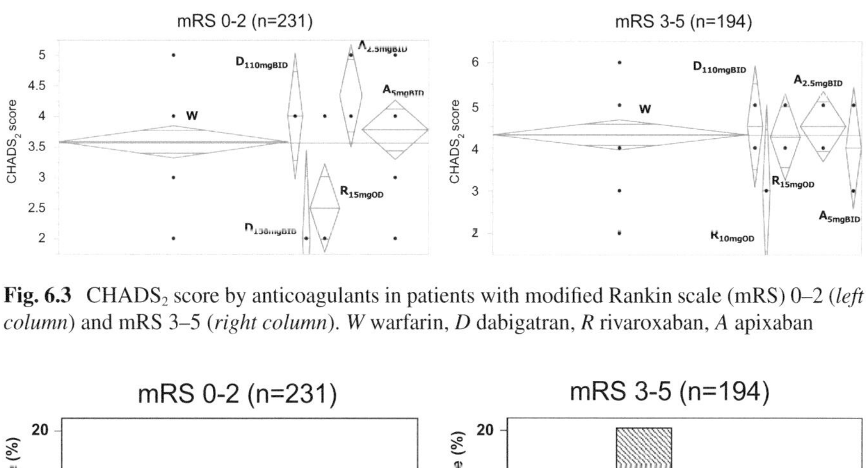

Fig. 6.3 $CHADS_2$ score by anticoagulants in patients with modified Rankin scale (mRS) 0–2 (*left column*) and mRS 3–5 (*right column*). *W* warfarin, *D* dabigatran, *R* rivaroxaban, *A* apixaban

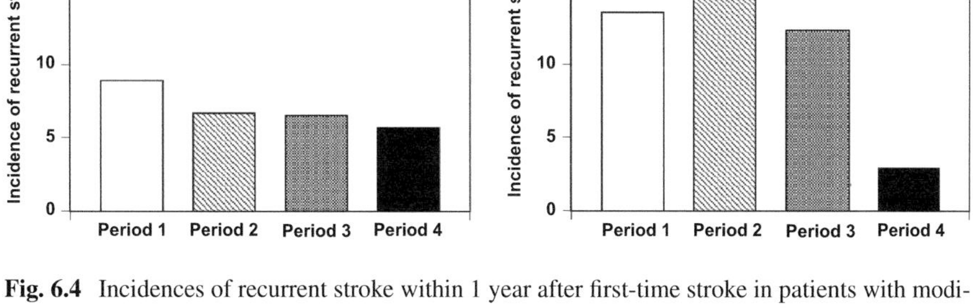

Fig. 6.4 Incidences of recurrent stroke within 1 year after first-time stroke in patients with modified Rankin scale (mRS) 0–2 (*left column*) and mRS 3–5 (*right column*)

Table 6.3 Incidence of recurrent stroke within 1 year after first-time stroke (%)

	W	$D_{110mgBID}$	$D_{150mgBID}$	R_{10mgOD}	R_{15mgOD}	$A_{2.5mgBID}$	A_{5mgBID}	Total
mRS 0–2								
Period 1	8.9							8.9
Period 2	6.7	7.7	0					6.7
Period 3	4.8	25.0	0	0	0			6.5
Period 4	8.6	0	0	N/A	0	0	0	5.7
mRS 3–5								
Period 1	13.5							13.5
Period 2	18.8	28.6	0					20.2
Period 3	13.5	0	N/A	0	0			12.3
Period 4	0	0	N/A	0	0	20.0	0	2.9

W warfarin, *D* dabigatran, *R* rivaroxaban, *A* apixaban, *mRS* modified Rankin scale

thus seemed to have a more significant impact on patients with severe disability than on those with mild disability. Interestingly, in Period 4, warfarin also reduced recurrent stroke compared to the other periods in patients with mRS 3–5.

6.3.3 Recurrent Ischemic Stroke

Mean durations of follow-up were 1109, 742, 642, and 202 days in Periods 1, 2, 3, and 4, respectively (Table 6.4). During the entire follow-up period, five recurrent cerebral infarcts occurred in patients who we had decided to treat with NOACs at the time of first-time discharge. All five cerebral infarcts occurred in patients treated with low-dose NOACs, with none in patients on standard-dose NOACs: three on low-dose dabigatran in Period 2, one on low-dose dabigatran in Period 2, and one on low-dose rivaroxaban in Period 3. In Period 4, no patient treated with NOACs experienced recurrent ischemic stroke.

In fact, four of the five cerebral infarcts did not represent pure recurrence. In two patients, cerebral infarcts occurred during unnecessarily long suspension of low-dose dabigatran due to other treatments in other departments. In one patient in whom dabigatran was inadequately reduced, the cerebral infarct occurred on regular medication. In one patient for whom anticoagulation had been changed from low-dose dabigatran to warfarin due to deterioration of renal dysfunction, the cerebral infarct occurred after cessation of dabigatran.

In the real world, a considerable amount of NOACs appear to be used at low dose despite the patient profile not complying with the criteria for dose reduction. Post-marketing surveillance has revealed that about 30 % of apixaban was inappropriately prescribed at low dose. However, evidence for the appropriateness of low-dose NOACs to achieve effective treatment seems somewhat fragile. RE-LY allocated patients equally to receive standard- or low-dose dabigatran, whereas far fewer patients were assigned to receive low-dose than standard-dose NOACs in ROCKET-AF, ARISTOTLE, and ENGAGE AF [1–4, 22].

We speculate that increases in the proportion of NOACs to warfarin as well as in the proportion of standard-dose to low-dose NOACs may have contributed to the improved treatment results in Period 4. Appropriate evaluation of hemorrhagic risk is definitely important, and low-dose NOACs may be safe in terms of hemorrhagic risk, but we believe that overestimation of the hemorrhagic risk and unwarranted dose reduction should be avoided.

6.3.4 Recurrent Hemorrhagic Stroke

One intracranial hemorrhage occurred in the patient treated with low-dose apixaban in Period 4 (Table 6.4). On the other hand, ten intracranial hemorrhages occurred in patients treated with warfarin during the entire period. Hematoma volume in the patient treated with apixaban was very small (1 mL) compared to the mean volume of the ten hematomas in patients treated with warfarin (52 mL). Two cases of gastrointestinal hemorrhage occurred among patients treated with low-dose dabigatran in Periods 2 and 4, whereas no cases of this complication were seen with standard-dose NOACs.

The intracranial vasculature is considered to be more vulnerable in Asian populations than in Western populations [23]. A multiethnic cohort of 18,867 patients hospitalized with first-time AF showed that the hazard ratio for intracranial hemorrhage during warfarin treatment is four times greater in Asians than in Whites [24]. The existence of microbleeds on T2* images was reported to increase the risk of intracranial hemorrhage 10.4-fold in an Asian population, compared to only 3.9-fold in a Western population [25].

Table 6.4 Number of patients with recurrent stroke during the entire follow-up period

	W	$D_{110mgBID}$	$D_{150mgBID}$	R_{10mgOD}	R_{15mgOD}	$A_{2.5mgBID}$	A_{5mgBID}	F/U (days)
Period 1	CI 34							1109 [448 ~ 1486]
	TIA 4							
	ICH 7							
	UK 1							
Period 2	CI 7	CI 3	0					742 [428 ~ 1101]
	TIA 2							
	ICH 2							
Period 3	CI 5	CI 1	0	CI 1	0			642 [104 ~ 739]
Period 4	CI 1	0	0	0	0	ICH 1	0	202 [146 ~ 373]
	ICH 1							

W warfarin, *D* dabigatran, *R* rivaroxaban, *A* apixaban, *F/U* follow-up, *CI* cerebral infarct, *TIA* transient ischemic attack, *ICH* intracranial hemorrhage

However, standard-dose NOACs seem suitable for Asian populations. A recent meta-analysis revealed that standard-dose NOACs were more effective in reducing stroke or systemic embolism in Asian populations than in non-Asian populations (odds ratio (OR) = 0.65, 95 % CI 0.52–0.83 versus OR = 0.85, 95 % CI 0.77–0.93; $p = 0.045$) and safer in Asian populations than in non-Asian populations in terms of major bleeding (OR = 0.57, 95 % CI 0.44–0.74 versus OR = 0.89, 95 % CI 0.76–1.04; $p = 0.004$), hemorrhagic stroke (OR = 0.32, 95 % CI 0.19–0.52 versus OR = 0.56, 95 % CI 0.44–0.70; $p = 0.046$), and gastrointestinal bleeding (OR = 0.79, 95 % CI 0.48–1.32 versus OR = 1.44, 95 % CI 1.12–1.85; $p = 0.041$), and low-dose NOACs were shown to perform similarly in both populations [26].

6.4 Conclusion

We believe that our principles in terms of choice of anticoagulants and dose selection have contributed to improved outcomes for secondary prevention of cerebral infarct in our hospital. Comparisons of current and previous treatment results may be helpful to self-check the validity of the decision-making process in individual hospitals and can contribute to improved outcomes for secondary prevention of cerebral infarct.

References

1. Connolly SJ, Ezekowitz MD, Yusuf S, Eikelboom J, Oldgren J, Parekh A, et al. Dabigatran versus warfarin in patients with atrial fibrillation. N Engl J Med. 2009;361(12):1139–51. doi:10.1056/NEJMoa0905561.
2. Giugliano RP, Ruff CT, Braunwald E, Murphy SA, Wiviott SD, Halperin JL, et al. Edoxaban versus warfarin in patients with atrial fibrillation. N Engl J Med. 2013;369(22):2093–104. doi:10.1056/NEJMoa1310907.
3. Granger CB, Alexander JH, McMurray JJ, Lopes RD, Hylek EM, Hanna M, et al. Apixaban versus warfarin in patients with atrial fibrillation. N Engl J Med. 2011;365(11):981–92. doi:10.1056/NEJMoa1107039.
4. Patel MR, Mahaffey KW, Garg J, Pan G, Singer DE, Hacke W, et al. Rivaroxaban versus warfarin in nonvalvular atrial fibrillation. N Engl J Med. 2011;365(10):883–91. doi:10.1056/NEJMoa1009638.
5. Ruff CT, Giugliano RP, Braunwald E, Hoffman EB, Deenadayalu N, Ezekowitz MD, et al. Comparison of the efficacy and safety of new oral anticoagulants with warfarin in patients with atrial fibrillation: a meta-analysis of randomised trials. Lancet. 2014;383(9921):955–62. doi:10.1016/S0140-6736(13)62343-0.
6. Gage BF, Waterman AD, Shannon W, Boechler M, Rich MW, Radford MJ. Validation of clinical classification schemes for predicting stroke: results from the National Registry of Atrial Fibrillation. JAMA. 2001;285(22):2864–70.
7. Pisters R, Lane DA, Nieuwlaat R, de Vos CB, Crijns HJ, Lip GY. A novel user-friendly score (HAS-BLED) to assess 1-year risk of major bleeding in patients with atrial fibrillation: the Euro Heart Survey. Chest. 2010;138(5):1093–100. doi:10.1378/chest.10-0134.

8. Apostolakis S, Lane DA, Guo Y, Buller H, Lip GY. Performance of the HEMORR(2)HAGES, ATRIA, and HAS-BLED bleeding risk-prediction scores in patients with atrial fibrillation undergoing anticoagulation: the AMADEUS (evaluating the use of SR34006 compared to warfarin or acenocoumarol in patients with atrial fibrillation) study. J Am Coll Cardiol. 2012;60(9):861–7. doi:10.1016/j.jacc.2012.06.019.
9. Roldan V, Marin F, Fernandez H, Manzano-Fernandez S, Gallego P, Valdes M, et al. Predictive value of the HAS-BLED and ATRIA bleeding scores for the risk of serious bleeding in a "real-world" population with atrial fibrillation receiving anticoagulant therapy. Chest. 2013;143(1):179–84. doi:10.1378/chest.12-0608.
10. Diener HC, Connolly SJ, Ezekowitz MD, Wallentin L, Reilly PA, Yang S, et al. Dabigatran compared with warfarin in patients with atrial fibrillation and previous transient ischaemic attack or stroke: a subgroup analysis of the RE-LY trial. Lancet Neurol. 2010;9(12):1157–63. doi:10.1016/S1474-4422(10)70274-X.
11. Group JCSJW. Guidelines for pharmacotherapy of atrial fibrillation (JCS 2013). Circ J. 2014;78(8):1997–2021.
12. Easton JD, Lopes RD, Bahit MC, Wojdyla DM, Granger CB, Wallentin L, et al. Apixaban compared with warfarin in patients with atrial fibrillation and previous stroke or transient ischaemic attack: a subgroup analysis of the ARISTOTLE trial. Lancet Neurol. 2012;11(6):503–11. doi:10.1016/S1474-4422(12)70092-3.
13. Gomez-Outes A, Terleira-Fernandez AI, Calvo-Rojas G, Suarez-Gea ML, Vargas-Castrillon E. Dabigatran, rivaroxaban, or apixaban versus warfarin in patients with nonvalvular atrial fibrillation: a systematic review and meta-analysis of subgroups. Thrombosis. 2013;2013:640723. doi:10.1155/2013/640723.
14. Hankey GJ, Patel MR, Stevens SR, Becker RC, Breithardt G, Carolei A, et al. Rivaroxaban compared with warfarin in patients with atrial fibrillation and previous stroke or transient ischaemic attack: a subgroup analysis of ROCKET AF. Lancet Neurol. 2012;11(4):315–22. doi:10.1016/S1474-4422(12)70042-X.
15. Harenberg J, Marx S, Wehling M. Head-to-head or indirect comparisons of the novel oral anticoagulants in atrial fibrillation: What's next? Thromb Haemost. 2012;108(3):407–9. doi:10.1160/TH12-07-0463.
16. Skjoth F, Larsen TB, Rasmussen LH. Indirect comparison studies--are they useful? Insights from the novel oral anticoagulants for stroke prevention in atrial fibrillation. Thromb Haemost. 2012;108(3):405–6. doi:10.1160/TH12-06-0438.
17. Harenberg J, Marx S, Diener HC, Lip GY, Marder VJ, Wehling M, et al. Comparison of efficacy and safety of dabigatran, rivaroxaban and apixaban in patients with atrial fibrillation using network meta-analysis. Int Angiol. 2012;31(4):330–9.
18. Lip GY, Larsen TB, Skjoth F, Rasmussen LH. Indirect comparisons of new oral anticoagulant drugs for efficacy and safety when used for stroke prevention in atrial fibrillation. J Am Coll Cardiol. 2012;60(8):738–46. doi:10.1016/j.jacc.2012.03.019.
19. Mantha S, Ansell J. An indirect comparison of dabigatran, rivaroxaban and apixaban for atrial fibrillation. Thromb Haemost. 2012;108(3):476–84. doi:10.1160/TH12-02-0093.
20. Savelieva I, Camm AJ. Practical considerations for using novel oral anticoagulants in patients with atrial fibrillation. Clin Cardiol. 2014;37(1):32–47. doi:10.1002/clc.22204.
21. Shields AM, Lip GY. Choosing the right drug to fit the patient when selecting oral anticoagulation for stroke prevention in atrial fibrillation. J Intern Med. 2015;278(1):1–18. doi:10.1111/joim.12360.
22. Hori M, Matsumoto M, Tanahashi N, Momomura S, Uchiyama S, Goto S, et al. Rivaroxaban vs. warfarin in Japanese patients with atrial fibrillation: the J-ROCKET AF study. Circ J. 2012;76(9):2104–11.
23. Ducrocq G, Bhatt DL, Labreuche J, Corbalan R, Porath A, Gao R, et al. Geographic differences in outcomes in outpatients with established atherothrombotic disease: results from the REACH registry. Eur J Prev Cardiol. 2014;21(12):1509–16. doi:10.1177/2047487313501278.

24. Shen AY, Yao JF, Brar SS, Jorgensen MB, Chen W. Racial/ethnic differences in the risk of intracranial hemorrhage among patients with atrial fibrillation. J Am Coll Cardiol. 2007;50(4):309–15. doi:10.1016/j.jacc.2007.01.098.
25. Charidimou A, Kakar P, Fox Z, Werring DJ. Cerebral microbleeds and recurrent stroke risk: systematic review and meta-analysis of prospective ischemic stroke and transient ischemic attack cohorts. Stroke. 2013;44(4):995–1001. doi:10.1161/STROKEAHA.111.000038.
26. Wang KL, Lip GY, Lin SJ, Chiang CE. Non-vitamin K antagonist oral anticoagulants for stroke prevention in Asian patients with nonvalvular atrial fibrillation: meta-analysis. Stroke. 2015;46(9):2555–61. doi:10.1161/STROKEAHA.115.009947.

Chapter 7
New Approaches for the Secondary Prevention of Cryptogenic Stroke Using Non-vitamin K Antagonist Oral Anticoagulants

Tomohisa Nezu and Yoshiki Yagita

Abstract Non-vitamin K antagonist oral anticoagulants (NOACs) were introduced to prevent systemic embolism in patients with non-valvular atrial fibrillation (AF), and the use of NOACs for secondary prevention of cardioembolic stroke in patients with AF has gradually increased. Recently, NOACs were also approved for the prevention for deep venous thrombosis. Therefore, ischemic stroke patients with paradoxical emboli who have right-to-left shunt (such as patent foramen ovale or pulmonary arteriovenous fistula) and deep venous thrombosis may be treated with NOACs. In addition, a new clinical concept, termed "Embolic Stroke of Undetermined Source" (ESUS), has recently been suggested. ESUS has been proposed as an indication for anticoagulation, because paroxysmal AF is a potential mechanism of stroke in ESUS patients. Some large randomized clinical trials have been initiated to determine whether NOACs are superior to antiplatelets for the prevention of recurrent stroke in patients with ESUS. In this review, we discuss the potential use of NOACs for secondary stroke prevention among ischemic stroke patients without AF, especially in patients with cryptogenic stroke.

Keywords Cryptogenic stroke • ESUS • NOACs • Anticoagulants

T. Nezu, MD, Ph.D. (✉)
Department of Clinical Neuroscience and Therapeutics, Hiroshima University, Graduate School of Biomedical & Health Sciences, Hiroshima, Japan

Department of Stroke Medicine, Kawasaki Medical School, Kurashiki, Japan
e-mail: dr.tom.n@gmail.com

Y. Yagita, MD, Ph.D.
Department of Stroke Medicine, Kawasaki Medical School, Kurashiki, Japan

M. Uno, K. Ogasawara (eds.), *Treatment of Non-vitamin K Antagonist Oral Anticoagulants*, DOI 10.1007/978-981-10-1878-7_7

7.1 Introduction

Non-vitamin K antagonist oral anticoagulants (NOACs) are at least equivalent to warfarin in terms of reducing the incidence of ischemic stroke and are superior to warfarin with regard to the risk of intracranial hemorrhage among patients with non-valvular atrial fibrillation (AF) [1–4]. NOACs are also useful for secondary stroke prevention in cardioembolic stroke patients with non-valvular AF. The use of NOACs for secondary prevention of cardioembolic stroke in patients with AF has gradually increased [5]. NOACs were originally used only in patients with non-valvular AF. Recently, four main NOACs (dabigatran, rivaroxaban, apixaban, and edoxaban) have been studied or approved for the treatment of deep venous thrombosis (DVT) and pulmonary embolism. Therefore, NOACs might be considered for use in the secondary prevention of stroke among ischemic stroke patients with DVT and paradoxical embolic stroke. In addition, anticoagulation therapy could be used in patients with cardioembolic stroke and AF as well as in patients with other stroke subtypes [6]. However, there is no evidence as to whether NOACs are useful for secondary stroke prevention among patients without AF.

Cryptogenic stroke (i.e., stroke of undetermined etiology) accounts for 20–40 % of all ischemic strokes [7, 8]. Patients with cryptogenic stroke have a high rate of stroke recurrence [9, 10]. However, the optimal antithrombotic strategy (e.g., antiplatelet drugs, anticoagulant drugs) in such patients remains unclear. In this review, we discuss the potential use of NOACs for secondary stroke prevention among ischemic stroke patients without AF, especially in patients with cryptogenic stroke.

7.2 Definition of Cryptogenic Ischemic Stroke or ESUS

Cryptogenic stroke generally refers to ischemic stroke of undetermined etiology and generally refers to a non-lacunar infarction occurring in the absence of a specific identifiable high-risk source of cardioembolism or large artery stenosis. However, the definition of cryptogenic stroke can vary according to the specific version of stroke subtype system [7]. In addition, the diagnosis of cryptogenic stroke depends on various diagnostic examinations, such as carotid ultrasonography, transthoracic echocardiography (TTE), transesophageal echocardiography (TEE), duration of continuous heart monitoring, frequency of Holter echocardiogram (ECG), and so on. Most cryptogenic stroke patients are likely to have strokes due to an embolic mechanism. Recently, a new clinical concept, termed “Embolic Stroke of Undetermined Source (ESUS),” was introduced [11]. The Cryptogenic Stroke/ESUS International Working Group has proposed that the patients with ESUS could gain more benefit from anticoagulation, especially anticoagulation with NOACs, when compared with antiplatelet therapy. The definition of ESUS is shown in Table 7.1. A physician can establish a diagnosis of ESUS after routine examinations. The potential causes among ESUS or cryptogenic stroke patients are shown in Table 7.2. Of these potential embolic sources, we focus on paroxysmal AF, paradoxical embolism, and aortic arch atheroma.

Table 7.1 Criteria for the diagnosis of Embolic Stroke of Undetermined Source (ESUS) using routine examinations[a] (Reproduced with permission from [11])

1.	Infarction detected by CT or MRI that is not lacunar[b]
2.	Absence of extracranial or intracranial atherosclerosis causing ≥50 % luminal stenosis in an artery supplying the area of recent brain ischemia
3.	No major-risk cardioembolic source[c]
4.	No other specific cause of stroke[d] identified

[a]Routine examinations are as follows: (1) brain computed tomography (CT) or magnetic resonance imaging (MRI), (2) 12-lead electrocardiogram, (3) precordial echocardiography, (4) cardiac monitoring for ≥24 h with automated rhythm detection, (5) imaging of both the extracranial and intracranial arteries supplying the area of brain ischemia (catheter, MR, or CT angiography, or cervical duplex plus transcranial Doppler ultrasonography)

[b]Lacunar defined as a subcortical infarct smaller than or equal to 1.5 cm (≤ 2.0 cm on MRI diffusion images) in the largest dimension, including on MRI diffusion images and in the distribution of the small, penetrating cerebral arteries

[c]Major-risk cardioembolic source: permanent or paroxysmal atrial fibrillation, sustained atrial flutter, intracardiac thrombus, prosthetic cardiac valve, atrial myxoma or other cardiac tumors, mitral stenosis, recent (< 4 weeks) myocardial infarction, left ventricular fraction less than 30 %, valvular vegetations, or infective endocarditis

[d]Other specific causes of stroke: arteritis, dissection, migraine/vasospasm, drug misuse, and so on

Table 7.2 Potential causes of Embolic Strokes of Undetermined Source (ESUS) or cryptogenic stroke

ESUS	
Potential cardioembolic source	
	Paroxysmal atrial fibrillation
	Mitral valve
	Myxomatous valvulopathy with prolapse
	Mitral annular calcification
	Aortic valve
	Aortic valve stenosis
	Calcific aortic valve
	Non-atrial fibrillation atrial dysrhythmias and stasis
	Atrial asystole and sick sinus syndrome
	Atrial high-rate episodes
	Atrial appendage stasis with reduced flow velocities or spontaneous echo-densities
	Atrial structural abnormalities
	Atrial septal aneurysm
	Chiari network
	Endomyocardial fibrosis
	Atrial myxoma
	Left ventricular hypertrabeculation
	Takotsubo cardiomyopathy
Paradoxical embolism (combined with deep venous thrombosis)	
	Patent foramen ovale
	Atrial septal defect
	Pulmonary arteriovenous fistula

(continued)

Table 7.2 (continued)

ESUS	
Arteriogenic emboli	
	Aortic arch atheroma
	Cerebral artery non-stenotic plaques with ulceration
Cancer associated	
	Covert nonbacterial thrombotic endocarditis
	Tumor emboli from occult cancer
Other specific causes of cryptogenic stroke	
Cerebral artery dissection	
Central nervous system vasculitis	
Fabry's disease	
Hypercoagulability	
	Antiphospholipid syndrome
	Hyperhomocysteinemia
	Nephrotic syndrome
	Antithrombin-III deficiency
	Protein-S deficiency
	Protein-C deficiency
	Factor XIII polymorphisms

Reproduced with permission from Ref. [11]

7.3 Paroxysmal AF

Paroxysmal AF is thought to be the most common potential mechanism of cryptogenic stroke or ESUS. Many studies have assessed various methods to detect paroxysmal AF in patients with ischemic stroke or cryptogenic stroke. In a 2007 systematic review, Liao et al. reported that screening consecutive ischemic stroke patients (n = 736) with 24–72 h continuous heart monitoring could identify new AF in approximately 5 % of cases [12]. A recent meta-analysis showed that the detection rate of new AF was 11.5 % among 5038 subjects in 32 studies and that new AF was detected in 15.9 % among 425 cryptogenic stroke patients [13]. However, the timing, duration, method of monitoring, and reporting of diagnostic criteria used for to diagnose paroxysmal AF or stroke subtype varied within this meta-analysis.

Recently, two randomized trials of prolonged monitoring to detect new paroxysmal AF after ischemic stroke have been conducted among patients with cryptogenic stroke [14, 15]. The Event Monitor Belt for Recording Atrial Fibrillation after a Cerebral Ischemic Event (EMBRACE) study was conducted to determine the diagnostic yield of 30-day cardiac rhythm monitoring versus repeat 24-h Holter ECG for detecting paroxysmal AF in cryptogenic stroke patients following routine diagnostic work-up, including an initial negative Holter ECG [15]. The primary outcome was the detection of one or more episodes of AF or atrial flutter lasting 30 s or more within 90 days. The EMBRACE trial showed that the new AF or atrial flutter was detected in 16.1 % of patients undergoing 30-day cardiac rhythm monitoring (n = 280) vs. 3.2 % of patients undergoing repeat 24-h Holter ECG (n = 277). The Cryptogenic Stroke and Underlying AF (CRYSTAL AF) trial was conducted to assess whether a long-term cardiac monitoring strategy via an implantable cardiac monitor (ICM) was superior to standard monitoring for detection of paroxysmal AF in cryptogenic stroke patients (14). AF was defined as an episode of irregular heart rhythm, without detectable p waves, of greater than 30 s. The primary outcome was the detection of AF within 6 months, and the secondary outcome was the detection of AF within 12 months. The investigators reported that AF was detected in 8.9 % of patients in the ICM group (n = 221) vs. in 1.4 % of patients in the standard monitoring group (n = 220) by 6 months and was detected in 12.4 % of patients in the ICM group vs. 2.0 % of patients in the standard monitoring group by 12 months. These clinical trials found that prolonged monitoring was superior to conventional follow-up for the detection of paroxysmal AF in patients with cryptogenic stroke. In addition, they provided further evidence that 10–20 % of cryptogenic stroke patients have underlying paroxysmal AF. Therefore, it is reasonable to consider anticoagulation therapy, especially NOACs, in patients with cryptogenic stroke or ESUS.

Aside from prolonged monitoring, there are various approaches to predict whether paroxysmal AF is the mechanism of cryptogenic stroke patients. For example, prolongation in the QTc or PR interval on ECG may indicate underlying paroxysmal AF [16, 17]. In addition, several studies showed that atrial premature beats on Holter ECG might predict paroxysmal AF in patients with cryptogenic stroke [18, 19]. TTE is also a useful modality to predict paroxysmal AF. Several studies found that left atrial size and left atrial function were associated with the detection of paroxysmal AF in patients with acute ischemic stroke [20]. In addition, biological markers, especially B-type natriuretic peptides, might be useful for the detection of paroxysmal AF in patients with cryptogenic stroke [21].

7.4 Paradoxical Embolism

Paradoxical embolism refers to the embolic entry of a venous thrombus into the systemic circulation through a right-to-left shunt (RLS) [22]. A patent foramen ovale (PFO) is a representative factor of RLS and is present in approximately 25–30 % of all patients with ischemic stroke [23]. A PFO can also be detected in 40–50 % of cryptogenic stroke patients [24, 25]. It is important to assess the size of the PFO and to assess for the presence of an atrial septal aneurysm and increased interatrial septal mobility in patients with ischemic stroke patients and PFO, because those factors might be associated with an increased risk of stroke recurrence [26, 27]. However, it remains controversial whether the presence of PFO is independently associated with the risk of recurrent stroke [23, 28].

Various methods, such as TTE, TEE, and transcranial Doppler (TCD) with a saline injection after the Valsalva maneuver, are used to detect RLS. TEE is considered the gold standard method to evaluate for PFO, because a TEE contrast study is more sensitive for the detection of PFO when compared with TCD and TTE [25]. In addition, TEE is also a useful method to assess PFO size as well as to assess for the presence of an arterial septal aneurysm and Chiari network. However, TEE is not a routine examination in patients with acute ischemic stroke, because it might be contraindicated due to decreased level of consciousness, bleeding tendency, and a risk of aspiration pneumonia. ESUS could be diagnosed after routine examinations without a TEE study as described above. Therefore, some patients with ESUS would be matched to the criteria for paradoxical embolism if they underwent the full work-up examinations.

There are insufficient data to establish whether anticoagulation is equivalent or superior to aspirin for secondary stroke prevention in patients with PFO. Therefore, according to recent American Heart Association/American Stroke Association guidelines, antiplatelet therapy is recommended for ischemic stroke patients with PFO who are not undergoing anticoagulation therapy (Class I, Level of Evidence B) [29]. On the other hand, these guidelines suggested that anticoagulation is indicated for patients with ischemic stroke who have both a PFO and a venous source of embolism (paradoxical embolism) (Class I, Level of Evidence A). However, the type of anticoagulation therapy, especially with regard to NOACs, was not described in these guidelines. Recently, four main NOACs (dabigatran, rivaroxaban, apixaban, and edoxaban) have been studied or approved for the treatment of deep venous thrombosis (DVT). However, there is no evidence as to the utility of NOACs for the secondary prevention of stroke in patients with paradoxical embolism. When considering the use of NOACs for this indication, one must consider the timing of initiation of NOACs after stroke onset. Early initiation of anticoagulation might be effective for the prevention of early stroke recurrence. However, early initiation of anticoagulation can also cause hemorrhagic transformation among patients with acute ischemic stroke, especially in those with large brain infarction. Clinical studies of patients with non-valvular AF found that NOACs should not be started within 7–14 days of a stroke onset [1–4]. Therefore, limited evidence exists with regard to the efficacy of NOACs for the secondary prevention of stroke, even in patients with non-valvular AF in acute stroke phase. Naturally, it is unclear whether NOACs are effective or safe in patients with paradoxical embolism who are in the acute stroke phase. Further, the optimal initial dose of NOACs in patients with paradoxical embolism is not clear. Studies have used different doses of NOACs (rivaroxaban and apixaban) in patients with acute DVT vs. in those with DVT [30]. Therefore, physicians should be careful with regard to the initial timing and initial dose when using NOACs for patients with paradoxical embolism.

7.5 Aortic Arch Atheroma

Aortic arch atheroma is thought to be a potential embolic source in patients with cryptogenic stroke or ESUS. Several studies showed that large aortic arch plaques (≥4 mm) were associated with an increased risk of ischemic stroke [31–33]. The French Study of Aortic Plaques in Stroke conducted TEE in 331 acute ischemic stroke patients and showed that large aortic arch plaque (≥4 mm) was an independent predictor of recurrent ischemic stroke after adjusting for the presence of carotid stenosis, AF, peripheral arterial disease, and other vascular risk factors (relative risk, 3.8; 95 % confidence interval [CI], 1.8–7.8; $P = 0.0012$) [33]. Complex morphological features of large plaques or mobile aortic plaques have also been shown to contribute to an increased risk of stroke [31, 34]. Although several studies showed that aortic plaques in the descending thoracic aorta might be a cause of cerebral embolism through retrograde aortic flow [35, 36], it remains controversial whether descending aortic plaques were associated with ischemic stroke [37].

The recently published American Heart Association/American Stroke Association guidelines recommended the use of antiplatelet therapy for ischemic stroke patients with evidence of aortic arch atheroma (Class I, Level of Evidence A). These guidelines show that the effectiveness of anticoagulation using warfarin compared with antiplatelet therapy to prevent the recurrence of stroke among patients with aortic arch plaques is unknown. (Class IIb, Level of Evidence C). Naturally, it is unclear whether NOACs is useful for the prevention of ischemic stroke among patients with aortic arch plaques. There is no evidence to support the use of dual antiplatelet therapy for the prevention of ischemic stroke among patients with aortic arch plaques. The Aortic Arch Related Cerebral Hazard (ARCH) trial was a prospective, randomized, open-label, blinded end point trial to compare the efficacy and safety of warfarin (internal normalized ration [INR] in the range of 2.0–3.0) versus clopidogrel (75 mg/day) plus aspirin (75 to 150 mg/day) for prevention of cardiovascular events [38]. Ischemic stroke patients with aortic arch plaques ≥4 mm and no other identified embolic source were recruited in this study. The investigators hypothesized that the combination of aspirin plus clopidogrel was 25 % superior to dose-adjusted warfarin with regard to the prevention of new cardiovascular events. However, the trial was stopped after 349 patients were randomized during a period of about 8 years. Cardiovascular events occurred in 7.6 % (13/172) of a patients in the aspirin plus clopidogrel and in 11.3 % (20/174) of patients in the warfarin (hazard ratio [HR], 0.76; 95 % CI, 0.36–1.61) after a median follow-up of 3.4 years. The hypothesis that dual antiplatelet therapy was superior to warfarin for the prevention of cardiovascular events among patients with aortic arch plaques was inconclusive, because of lack of statistical power.

7.6 Clinical Studies of Secondary Prevention of Stroke in Patients with Cryptogenic Stroke

The Warfarin-Aspirin Recurrent Stroke Study (WARSS) was conducted to investigate whether warfarin was superior to aspirin for the prevention of recurrent stroke in patients with non-cardioembolic stroke [39]. The warfarin doses were adjusted to achieve and maintain an INR in the range of 1.4–2.8. However, there was no difference between aspirin and warfarin in the prevention of recurrent ischemic stroke or death or in the rate of major hemorrhage over 2 years. In addition, warfarin was not superior to aspirin with regard to recurrent events or death among the subgroup of patients with cryptogenic stroke. The Patent Foramen Ovale in Cryptogenic Stroke Study (PICSS) which was a sub-study of the WARSS that sought to define the rate of recurrent stroke or death in stroke patients with or without a TEE-defined PFO who were randomly assigned to warfarin or aspirin in a double-blind study design [23]. There was no significant difference in the time to recurrent ischemic stroke or death between patients with vs. without PFO. In addition, there was no significant difference in the time to the recurrent ischemic stroke or death between patients treated with warfarin and those treated with aspirin among patients with PFO. Another sub-study of the PICCS investigated the association between aortic arch atheroma and recurrent stroke events [31]. Large aortic plaques (≥4 mm) were significantly associated with recurrent ischemic stroke or death (HR, 2.12; 95 % CI, 1.04–4.32), especially with regard to plaque with complex morphology (HR, 2.55; 95 % CI, 1.10–5.89), which is consistent with results from previous studies [31, 33, 34]. However, there was no interaction between warfarin and large aortic plaques with regard to the risk of events. Subjects in the WARRS or PICCS studies were recruited during the period between 1993 and 2000. On the other hand, the ARCH study, which was designed to clarify whether dual antiplatelet therapy was superior to warfarin for the prevention of cardiovascular events among patients with aortic arch plaques (described above), was conducted during the period between 2002 and 2010 [38]. Table 7.3 shows the summary of results from the WARSS, PICCS, and ARCH studies. The event rate among patients in the ARCH study was lower than that among patients with large plaques in the PICCS study. One of the reasons for this finding might be the different medical management use to address vascular risk factors (such as statin therapy, antihypertensive agents, and so on). In the future, when trying to determine the optimal antithrombotic therapy (anticoagulation vs. antiplatelet therapy) to prevent recurrent stroke among patients with cryptogenic stroke, investigators should also refer another medical management to control the vascular risk factors.

The concept of ESUS was proposed to clarify whether patients with potential embolic source could gain more benefit from anticoagulation, especially NOACs, than from antiplatelet therapy. Today, two large randomized clinical trials to determine whether NOACs is superior to aspirin for prevention of recurrent stroke among patients with ESUS are planned. The Randomized, double-blind, Evaluation in secondary Stroke Prevention comparing the EfficaCy and safety of the oral Thrombin inhibitor dabigatran etexilate vs. acetylsalicylic acid in patients with Embolic Stroke of Undetermined Source (RESPECT ESUS) investigators plans to randomize 6000 patients with ESUS to dabigatran (110 mg or 150 mg twice daily) vs. aspirin (100 mg once daily) for the purposes of prevention of recurrent stroke (ischemic, hemorrhagic, or unspecified) over a period of 3 years (NCT02239120) [40]. The Rivaroxaban vs. Aspirin in Secondary Prevention of Stroke and Prevention of Systemic Embolism in Patients with Recent Embolic Stroke of Undetermined Source (NAVIGATE ESUS) investigators plan to randomize 7060 patients to rivaroxaban (15 mg once daily) vs. aspirin (100 mg once daily) over a period of 3 years, and the primary outcomes are time to recurrent stroke (ischemic, hemorrhagic, or unspecified), systemic embolism, or major bleeding (NCT02313909).

Table 7.3 Summary of the Warfarin-Aspirin Recurrent Stroke Study (WARSS), Patent Foramen Ovale in Cryptogenic Stroke Study (PICCS), and Aortic Arch Related Cerebral Hazard (ARCH) studies. Primary end points are recurrent ischemic stroke or death in the WARSS and PICCS studies and recurrent stroke (ischemic or hemorrhagic), myocardial infarction, peripheral embolism, or vascular death in the ARCH study

Study	Subjects	Follow-up	Group	Primary end points	Hazard ratio (95 % confidence interval)	P value
WARSS 2001	Non-cardioembolic stroke (n = 2206)	2 years	Warfarin, n = 1103	17.8 %	1.13 (0.92–1.38)[a]	0.25
			Aspirin, n = 1103	16.0 %		
	Cryptogenic stroke (n = 576)	2 years	Warfarin, n = 281	15.0 %	0.92 (0.61–1.39)[a]	0.68
			Aspirin, n = 295	16.5 %		
PICSS 2002	Patients underwent TEE in WARSS	2 years	With PFO, n = 203	14.8 %	0.96 (0.62–1.48)[b]	0.84
			Without PFO, n = 398	15.4 %		
	Patients with PFO in PICSS	2 years	Warfarin, n = 97	16.5 %	1.29 (0.63–2.64)[a]	0.49
			Aspirin, n = 106	13.2 %		
PICSS 2009	Patients underwent TEE in WARSS (n = 516)	2 years	Large plaques, n = 101	26.7 %	2.12 (1.04–4.32)[c]	Data not shown
			Small plaques, n = 236	16.5 %		
			No plaques, n = 179	10.1 %		
ARCH 2014	Patients with large plaques (n = 349)	3.4 years	Aspirin+clopidogrel, n = 172	7.6 %	0.76 (0.36–1.61)[d]	0.5
			Warfarin, n = 177	11.3 %		

[a]Hazard ratio (HR) for warfarin as compared with aspirin
[b]HR for patients with PFO as compared with those without
[c]HR for large plaques as compared with no plaques
[d]HR for aspirin+clopidogrel compared with warfarin
TEE transesophageal echocardiography
PFO patent foramen ovale

7.7 Potential Use of NOACs for Secondary Stroke Prevention in Patients with Other Mechanisms of Ischemic Stroke

7.7.1 Cerebral Artery Dissection

The potential use of NOACs is also being considered in patients with other mechanisms of ischemic stroke. The Cervical Artery Dissection In Stroke Study (CADISS) was established to compare the efficacy of antiplatelet drugs vs. anticoagulation for the prevention of recurrent stroke in patients with carotid and vertebral artery dissection [41]. A total of 250 patients were recruited, and the primary end point was ipsilateral stroke or death within 3 months of randomization. Stroke or death occurred in three (2 %) of 126 patients receiving antiplatelet drugs vs. in one (1 %) of 124 patients receiving anticoagulants ($P = 0.63$). Early stroke recurrence is very rare in ischemic stroke patients with cerebral artery dissection. Therefore, the comparative efficacy of warfarin vs. antiplatelet drugs in ischemic stroke patients with cerebral artery dissection remains unknown. Recently, one single-center retrospective study showed that NOACs may be a reasonable alternative for the management of cervical artery dissection [42]. Clinical trials to clarify the optimal antithrombotic medications (NOACs vs. antiplatelet use) for secondary stroke prevention among patients with cerebral artery dissection will need a very large sample size.

7.7.2 Antiphospholipid Syndrome

Antiphospholipid syndrome (APS) is diagnosed in a patient with venous or arterial thrombosis who has persistent antiphospholipid antibodies. Antiphospholipid antibodies are thought to be risk factors for ischemic stroke in young patients as well as in elderly patients. Anticoagulation therapy with warfarin is currently the mainstay of treatment of thrombotic APS. Recent guidelines recommended that the target INR for warfarin therapy should be 2.5 (range, 2.0–3.0) for APS patients, especially in patients with a history of venous thrombosis [43]. On the other hand, there is no evidence as to whether NOACs are useful for the secondary prevention of thrombotic events in APS patients. The Rivaroxaban in AntiPhospholipid Syndrome (RAPS) trial is a prospective randomized controlled trial that will evaluate whether rivaroxaban is non-inferior to warfarin (target INR range, 2.0–3.0) for the prevention of thromboembolic events and major bleeding and maintenance of quality of life in APS patients with venous thromboembolism (NCT02116036) [44].

7.8 Conclusions

The efficacy and safety of NOACs for secondary stroke prevention have recently been studied in patients with various types of ischemic stroke [45]. Paroxysmal AF is thought to be the most frequent potential mechanism of stroke in patients with cryptogenic stroke or ESUS. Therefore, NOACs may be a reasonable option for secondary stroke prevention in those patients. A conclusive determination of the utility of NOACs for the secondary prevention of ischemic stroke in patients with cryptogenic stroke or ESUS will be determined in several large randomized trials.

References

1. Patel MR, Mahaffey KW, Garg J, Pan G, Singer DE, Hacke W, et al. Rivaroxaban versus warfarin in nonvalvular atrial fibrillation. N Engl J Med. 2011;365(10):883–91.

2. Connolly SJ, Ezekowitz MD, Yusuf S, Eikelboom J, Oldgren J, Parekh A, et al. Dabigatran versus warfarin in patients with atrial fibrillation. N Engl J Med. 2009;361(12):1139–51.
3. Granger CB, Alexander JH, McMurray JJ, Lopes RD, Hylek EM, Hanna M, et al. Apixaban versus warfarin in patients with atrial fibrillation. N Engl J Med. 2011;365(11):981–92.
4. Giugliano RP, Ruff CT, Braunwald E, Murphy SA, Wiviott SD, Halperin JL, et al. Edoxaban versus warfarin in patients with atrial fibrillation. N Engl J Med. 2013;369(22):2093–104.
5. Toyoda K, Arihiro S, Todo K, Yamagami H, Kimura K, Furui E, et al. Trends in oral anticoagulant choice for acute stroke patients with nonvalvular atrial fibrillation in Japan: the SAMURAI-NVAF study. Int J Stroke. 2015;10(6):836–42.
6. Furie KL, Kasner SE, Adams RJ, Albers GW, Bush RL, Fagan SC, et al. Guidelines for the prevention of stroke in patients with stroke or transient ischemic attack: a guideline for healthcare professionals from the American Heart Association/American Stroke Association. Stroke. 2011;42(1):227–76.
7. Marnane M, Duggan CA, Sheehan OC, Merwick A, Hannon N, Curtin D, et al. Stroke subtype classification to mechanism-specific and undetermined categories by TOAST, A-S-C-O, and causative classification system: direct comparison in the North Dublin population stroke study. Stroke. 2010;41(8):1579–86.
8. Grau AJ, Weimar C, Buggle F, Heinrich A, Goertler M, Neumaier S, et al. Risk factors, outcome, and treatment in subtypes of ischemic stroke: the German stroke data bank. Stroke. 2001;32(11):2559–66.
9. Bang OY, Lee PH, Joo SY, Lee JS, Joo IS, Huh K. Frequency and mechanisms of stroke recurrence after cryptogenic stroke. Ann Neurol. 2003;54(2):227–34.
10. Bal S, Patel SK, Almekhlafi M, Modi J, Demchuk AM, Coutts SB. High rate of magnetic resonance imaging stroke recurrence in cryptogenic transient ischemic attack and minor stroke patients. Stroke. 2012;43(12):3387–8.
11. Hart RG, Diener HC, Coutts SB, Easton JD, Granger CB, O'Donnell MJ, et al. Embolic strokes of undetermined source: the case for a new clinical construct. Lancet Neurol. 2014;13(4):429–38.
12. Liao J, Khalid Z, Scallan C, Morillo C, O'Donnell M. Noninvasive cardiac monitoring for detecting paroxysmal atrial fibrillation or flutter after acute ischemic stroke: a systematic review. Stroke. 2007;38(11):2935–40.
13. Kishore A, Vail A, Majid A, Dawson J, Lees KR, Tyrrell PJ, et al. Detection of atrial fibrillation after ischemic stroke or transient ischemic attack: a systematic review and meta-analysis. Stroke. 2014;45(2):520–6.
14. Sanna T, Diener HC, Passman RS, Di Lazzaro V, Bernstein RA, Morillo CA, et al. Cryptogenic stroke and underlying atrial fibrillation. N Engl J Med. 2014;370(26):2478–86.
15. Gladstone DJ, Spring M, Dorian P, Panzov V, Thorpe KE, Hall J, et al. Atrial fibrillation in patients with cryptogenic stroke. N Engl J Med. 2014;370(26):2467–77.
16. Thijs VN, Brachmann J, Morillo CA, Passman RS, Sanna T, Bernstein RA, et al. Predictors for atrial fibrillation detection after cryptogenic stroke: results from CRYSTAL AF. Neurology. 2016;86(3):261–9.
17. Hoshino T, Nagao T, Shiga T, Maruyama K, Toi S, Mizuno S, et al. Prolonged QTc interval predicts poststroke paroxysmal atrial fibrillation. Stroke. 2015;46(1):71–6.
18. Gladstone DJ, Dorian P, Spring M, Panzov V, Mamdani M, Healey JS, et al. Atrial premature beats predict atrial fibrillation in cryptogenic stroke: results from the EMBRACE trial. Stroke. 2015;46(4):936–41.
19. Kochhäuser S, Dechering DG, Dittrich R, Reinke F, Ritter MA, Ramtin S, et al. Supraventricular premature beats and short atrial runs predict atrial fibrillation in continuously monitored patients with cryptogenic stroke. Stroke. 2014;45(3):884–6.
20. Stahrenberg R, Edelmann F, Haase B, Lahno R, Seegers J, Weber-Krüger M, et al. Transthoracic echocardiography to rule out paroxysmal atrial fibrillation as a cause of stroke or transient ischemic attack. Stroke. 2011;42(12):3643–5.

21. Shibazaki K, Kimura K, Fujii S, Sakai K, Iguchi Y. Brain natriuretic peptide levels as a predictor for new atrial fibrillation during hospitalization in patients with acute ischemic stroke. Am J Cardiol. 2012;109(9):1303–7.
22. Loscalzo J. Paradoxical embolism: clinical presentation, diagnostic strategies, and therapeutic options. Am Heart J. 1986;112(1):141–5.
23. Homma S, Sacco RL, Di Tullio MR, Sciacca RR, Mohr JP. Investigators PiCSSP. Effect of medical treatment in stroke patients with patent foramen ovale: patent foramen ovale in cryptogenic stroke study. Circulation. 2002;105(22):2625–31.
24. Handke M, Harloff A, Olschewski M, Hetzel A, Geibel A. Patent foramen ovale and cryptogenic stroke in older patients. N Engl J Med. 2007;357(22):2262–8.
25. Homma S, Sacco RL. Patent foramen ovale and stroke. Circulation. 2005;112(7):1063–72.
26. Schuchlenz HW, Weihs W, Horner S, Quehenberger F. The association between the diameter of a patent foramen ovale and the risk of embolic cerebrovascular events. Am J Med. 2000;109(6):456–62.
27. Mas JL, Arquizan C, Lamy C, Zuber M, Cabanes L, Derumeaux G, et al. Recurrent cerebrovascular events associated with patent foramen ovale, atrial septal aneurysm, or both. N Engl J Med. 2001;345(24):1740–6.
28. Serena J, Marti-Fàbregas J, Santamarina E, Rodríguez JJ, Perez-Ayuso MJ, Masjuan J, et al. Recurrent stroke and massive right-to-left shunt: results from the prospective Spanish multicenter (CODICIA) study. Stroke. 2008;39(12):3131–6.
29. Kernan WN, Ovbiagele B, Black HR, Bravata DM, Chimowitz MI, Ezekowitz MD, et al. Guidelines for the prevention of stroke in patients with stroke and transient ischemic attack: a guideline for healthcare professionals from the American Heart Association/American Stroke Association. Stroke. 2014;45(7):2160–236.
30. Wells PS, Forgie MA, Rodger MA. Treatment of venous thromboembolism. JAMA. 2014;311(7):717–28.
31. Di Tullio MR, Russo C, Jin Z, Sacco RL, Mohr JP, Homma S, et al. Aortic arch plaques and risk of recurrent stroke and death. Circulation. 2009;119(17):2376–82.
32. Amarenco P, Cohen A, Tzourio C, Bertrand B, Hommel M, Besson G, et al. Atherosclerotic disease of the aortic arch and the risk of ischemic stroke. N Engl J Med. 1994;331(22):1474–9.
33. The French Study of Aortic Plaques in Stroke Group. Atherosclerotic disease of the aortic arch as a risk factor for recurrent ischemic stroke. N Engl J Med. 1996;334(19):1216–21.
34. Di Tullio MR, Sacco RL, Gersony D, Nayak H, Weslow RG, Kargman DE, et al. Aortic atheromas and acute ischemic stroke: a transesophageal echocardiographic study in an ethnically mixed population. Neurology. 1996;46(6):1560–6.
35. Chhabra L, Niroula R, Phadke J, Spodick DH. Retrograde embolism from the descending thoracic aorta causing stroke: an underappreciated clinical condition. Indian Heart J. 2013;65(3):319–22.
36. Harloff A, Simon J, Brendecke S, Assefa D, Helbing T, Frydrychowicz A, et al. Complex plaques in the proximal descending aorta: an underestimated embolic source of stroke. Stroke. 2010;41(6):1145–50.
37. Katsanos AH, Giannopoulos S, Kosmidou M, Voumvourakis K, Parissis JT, Kyritsis AP, et al. Complex atheromatous plaques in the descending aorta and the risk of stroke: a systematic review and meta-analysis. Stroke. 2014;45(6):1764–70.
38. Amarenco P, Davis S, Jones EF, Cohen AA, Heiss WD, Kaste M, et al. Clopidogrel plus aspirin versus warfarin in patients with stroke and aortic arch plaques. Stroke. 2014;45(5):1248–57.
39. Mohr JP, Thompson JL, Lazar RM, Levin B, Sacco RL, Furie KL, et al. A comparison of warfarin and aspirin for the prevention of recurrent ischemic stroke. N Engl J Med. 2001;345(20):1444–51.
40. Diener HC, Easton JD, Granger CB, Cronin L, Duffy C, Cotton D, et al. Design of Randomized, double-blind, Evaluation in secondary Stroke Prevention comparing the EfficaCy and safety of the oral Thrombin inhibitor dabigatran etexilate vs. acetylsalicylic acid in patients with

Embolic Stroke of Undetermined Source (RE-SPECT ESUS). Int J Stroke. 2015;10(8):1309–12.
41. Markus HS, Hayter E, Levi C, Feldman A, Venables G, Norris J, et al. Antiplatelet treatment compared with anticoagulation treatment for cervical artery dissection (CADISS): a randomised trial. Lancet Neurol. 2015;14(4):361–7.
42. Caprio FZ, Bernstein RA, Alberts MJ, Curran Y, Bergman D, Korutz AW, et al. Efficacy and safety of novel oral anticoagulants in patients with cervical artery dissections. Cerebrovasc Dis. 2014;38(4):247–53.
43. Keeling D, Mackie I, Moore GW, Greer IA, Greaves M. Haematology BCfSi. Guidelines on the investigation and management of antiphospholipid syndrome. Br J Haematol. 2012;157(1):47–58.
44. Cohen H, Doré CJ, Clawson S, Hunt BJ, Isenberg D, Khamashta M, et al. Rivaroxaban in antiphospholipid syndrome (RAPS) protocol: a prospective, randomized controlled phase II/III clinical trial of rivaroxaban versus warfarin in patients with thrombotic antiphospholipid syndrome, with or without SLE. Lupus. 2015;24(10):1087–94.
45. Yaghi S, Kamel H, Elkind MS. Potential new uses of non-vitamin K antagonist oral anticoagulants to treat and prevent stroke. Neurology. 2015;85(12):1078–84.

Chapter 8
Putaminal Hemorrhage in Patients with Oral Anticoagulants: Course of Treatment and Results of Endoscopic Evacuation

Nobuhisa Matsushita and Masaaki Uno

Abstract With the aging of the population, the use of oral anticoagulants (ACs) has been increasing. Intracerebral hemorrhage (ICH) is a potentially fatal complication during use of ACs. Surgical evacuation of hematoma located in the deep cerebrum is controversial, but with the continued evolution of endoscopy, surgical evacuation of putaminal hemorrhage is becoming safer and less invasive.

Methods: We retrospectively reviewed the medical records of all cases of AC-related ICH treated at Kawasaki Medical School Hospital during the 10-year period from 2004 to 2015.

Result: A total of 1100 cases of spontaneous ICH were treated at our institution during the study period, with 9.7 % (107 cases) related to oral ACs. We identified 359 patients with putaminal hemorrhage, of whom 7.0 % (25 patients) showed AC-related ICH. Surgical evacuation was considered contraindicated for 20 patients with AC-related putaminal hemorrhage due to insufficient or excessive hematoma volume. Surgical evacuation was performed for five cases, including two cases with expanding hematoma. In the most recent 3 years, we performed endoscopic evacuation for 32 patients with putaminal hemorrhage, including 5AC-related cases. Patients on ACs were older and showed a larger volume of hematoma. In AC-related ICH, hematoma growth was seen twice as often as in ICH unrelated to AC. The evacuation rate of hematoma was over 95 % for both types, with no rebleeding in any cases. The rate of poor outcomes (modified Rankin scale score, 5–6) at 3 months was 40 % (2/5) for AC-related ICH and 31.25 % (10/32) for ICH unrelated to ACs.

Conclusion: Even under oral anticoagulation, with suitable reversal of coagulability, endoscopic evacuation could be performed safely.

Keywords Putaminal hemorrhage • Oral anticoagulants • Endoscopic evacuation

---

N. Matsushita, M.D., Ph.D. (✉) • M. Uno, M.D., Ph.D.
Department of Neurosurgery, Kawasaki Medical School, 577 Matsushima, Kurashiki, Okayama 701-0192, Japan
e-mail: nobuhisama@gmail.com

M. Uno, K. Ogasawara (eds.), *Treatment of Non-vitamin K Antagonist Oral Anticoagulants*, DOI 10.1007/978-981-10-1878-7_8

8.1 Introduction

With the aging of the population, the use of oral anticoagulants (ACs) to prevent cardioembolic stroke has been increasing. For decades, vitamin K antagonists (VKAs) have been the most widely used ACs for stroke prophylaxis in patients with nonvalvular atrial fibrillation (NVAF). However, the efficacy of VKAs is markedly influenced by the time in therapeutic range, which requires regular monitoring of blood levels. Intracerebral hemorrhage (ICH) is responsible for most deaths caused by bleeding complications during long-term AC use. ICH during anticoagulation with VKAs accounts for 10–25 % of all occurrences if ICH [1]. Past reports have found that use of VKAs immediately prior to ICH was independently associated with increased early mortality, while normalization of coagulation parameters failed to affect outcomes [2, 3]. Conversely, a recent report found that pretreatment with oral AC represented an independent predictor of inhospital mortality but only among patients treated conservatively [4]. This suggests that therapeutic efforts to rapidly reverse coagulopathy and evacuate hematoma may represent a lifesaving treatment even in patients on ACs.

Large ICH should undoubtedly be evacuated if the life of the patient is to be saved. However, the role of surgical evacuation in the treatment of supratentorial ICH is much less established, and the decision of whether to evacuate these hematomas remains controversial. According to randomized controlled trials, traditional open craniotomy and hematoma evacuation for ICH are not beneficial in patients with ICH who are not in need of emergent lifesaving [5, 6]. However, with the evolution of endoscopy and hemostatic agents, surgical evacuation of ICH even in deep locations continues to become safer and less invasive.

This retrospective analysis reviewed the clinical course of patients with putaminal hemorrhage, which represents the most common form of ICH related to ACs, and evaluated the influence of VKAs on the results of endoscopic evacuation as a minimally invasive surgery.

8.2 Patients and Methods

8.2.1 Patients

Between April 2004 and March 2015, a total of 1100 patients with spontaneous ICH were brought to our institution. A summary of this cohort is shown in Table 8.1. Of these, 107 cases (9.7 %) were related to oral AC. During the same period, we treated 359 patients with putaminal hemorrhage. In this sub-cohort, 147 cases (40.9 %) received surgical evacuation. Surgical indications were in line with the Japanese guidelines for the management of stroke [18, 19]. Hematoma volume in each case was calculated as maximum diameter × diameter perpendicular to maximum diameter × height × 1/2, as an approximation using data from computed tomography

Table 8.1 Summary of patients treated between April 2004 and March 2015

			Anticoagulants	No anticoagulants
Spontaneous ICH		1100	107/1100	993
			9.7 %	
Putaminal hemorrhage		359	25/359	334
			7.0 %	
Surgical evacuation		147		
	Endoscope	101	5/147	96
	Craniotomy	46	0	46
Conservative		212	20	192

Table 8.2 Summary of cases with putaminal hemorrhage treated by endoscopic evacuation between January 2011 and March 2015

Putaminal hemorrhage treated by evacuation		Anticoagulants	No anticoagulants
Endoscope	37	5	32

(CT). From 2006, we selected endoscopic evacuation as the first-choice surgical treatment. The technical procedures are described in detail in the next section. Between January 2011 and March 2015, we established a surgical technique for the endoscope and performed endoscopic evacuation for 32 patients with putaminal hemorrhage, including five cases related to use of oral ACs (Table 8.2).

8.2.2 Surgical Procedure

The procedure needed to be performed in the acute stage. The target volume for hematoma to be eligible for evacuation was ≥31 ml, as this size facilitated simple access to the hematoma cavity. The entry site was placed 80–125 mm superior to a point 27 mm lateral to the nasion, as reported by Yokosuka et al. [7] After the sheath reached the surface of the hematoma, the endoscope was introduced. We used a 4-mm rigid endoscope (Karl Storz, Tuttlingen, Germany), Neuroport transparent sheath (Olympus, Tokyo, Japan), and irrigation aspirator (Fujita Medical Instruments, Tokyo, Japan). The hematoma was evacuated from the upper surface to the deep side. While advancing the endoscope, the transparent sheath allowed clear visualization of the border between the hematoma and brain parenchyma. When intraoperative hemorrhage occurred, the operating field was kept clear with repeated irrigation and continuous suction. This technique was reported by Nagasaka et al. [8] Irrigation and suction volumes were balanced, so identification and coagulation of the bleeding artery could be performed under clear visualization. Sufficient irrigation required not only manipulation of the irrigation channel of the irrigation aspirator but also assistance by manual injection of saline. Oozing in the hematoma cavity was treated using oxidized cellulose (Surgicel; Ethicon, Johnson & Johnson, New Brunswick, NJ). Finally, we confirmed a clear view of the hematoma cavity through the transparent sheath and finished the procedure.

8.3 Results

8.3.1 Course of Putaminal Hemorrhage with Anticoagulation

Between April 2004 and March 2015, we treated 359 patients with putaminal hemorrhage. Within this cohort, 25 cases (7.0 %) showed AC-related ICH. Mean prothrombin time-international normalized ratio (PT-INR) on admission of ICH patients who had been receiving VKAs was 2.3 ± 0.76, and 84.0 % (21/25) showed PT-INR <3.0. Only three patients (12 %) showed a hematoma volume suitable for surgical evacuation on initial CT examination. Eleven patients with hematoma volume > 100 ml on initial examination were excluded from surgical evacuation. Only one patient (1/11 with hematoma volume > 100 ml) underwent surgical evacuation because some of them survive. Five (45.5 %) of the 11 patients with hematoma volume > 100 ml were on hemodialysis. On the other hand, nine patients showed a hematoma volume < 30 ml at initial examination and were treated conservatively. Surgical evacuation was necessary due to expansion of the hematoma in two cases (22.2 %). Surgical evacuation was performed for five cases (20 %). All cases in which surgical evacuation was performed had been treated using VKAs. Outcome at 3 months was modified Rankin scale (mRS) four in three patients and mRS five in one patient, while one patient died in hospital. These results are shown in Fig. 8.1.

8.3.2 Results for Endoscopic Evacuation of Putaminal Hemorrhage with and Without ACs

We divided patients with putaminal hemorrhage who underwent endoscopic evacuation between 2011 and 2015 into subgroups treated with AC (AC group) or without AC (n-AC group) and compared these cohorts. Median age tended to be higher for the AC group (67.0 ± 10.6 years) than for the n-AC group (61.4 ± 11.3 years; n.s.). Mean hematoma volume also tended to be higher for the AC group (77 ± 28.1 ml) than for the n-AC group (62.4 ± 25.9 ml; n.s.). Median time from onset to surgery was 8.1 h for the AC group and 5.1 h for the n-AC group. Expansion of hematoma was seen in one case (20 %) in the AC group and three cases (9.4 %) in the n-AC group. Hematoma growth was twice as common for AC-related ICH than for ICH unrelated to AC, although again the difference was not significant. Median operative time was 90.8 ± 31.0 min in the AC group and 70.1 ± 27.7 min in the n-AC group, with patients on ACs tending to require longer to finish the procedure (n.s.). Evacuation rate for the hematoma was >95 % in both groups, and no cases of rebleeding were encountered. The rate of poor outcome (mRS 5–6) at 3 months was 40 % (2/5) in the AC group and 31.25 % (10/32) in the n-AC group, showing no significant difference. The results are shown in Table 8.3, and a representative case of growing hematoma that was evacuated endoscopically is shown in Fig. 8.2.

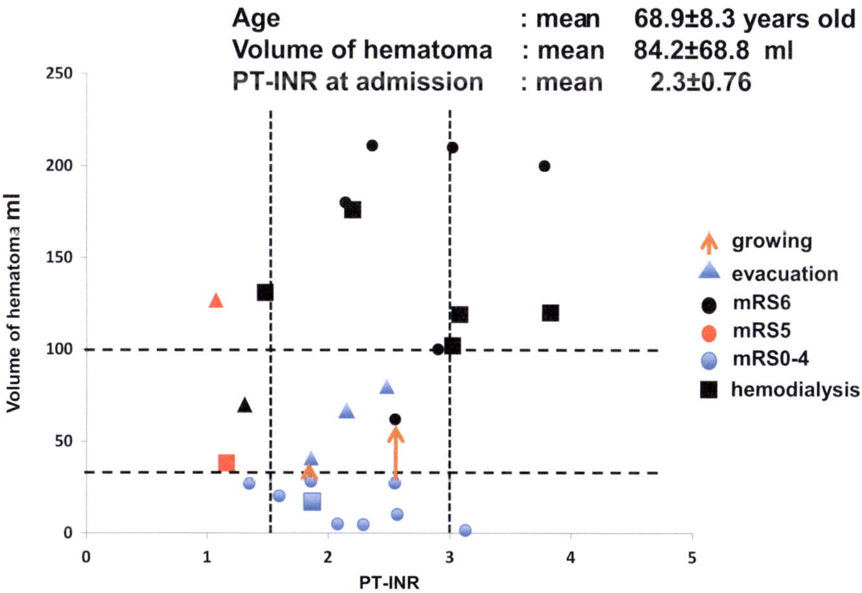

Fig. 8.1 Twenty-five cases of putaminal hemorrhage with VKAs

Table 8.3 Summary of patients with putaminal hemorrhage treated by endoscopic evacuation between January 2011 and March 2015

	n–AC ($n = 32$)	AC ($n = 5$)
Age (years)	61.4 ± 11.3	67.0 ± 10.6
Hematoma volume (ml)	62.4 ± 25.9	77 ± 28.1
Period from onset to evacuation (h)	5.1	8.1
Growing hematomas (n, %)	3 (9.4 %)	1 (20 %)
Operation time (min)	70.1 ± 27.7	90.8 ± 31.0
Evacuation rate (%)	>95 %	>95 %
Rebleeding episodes (n)	0	0
Poor outcome (mRS 5–6)	31.25 % (10/32)	40 % (2/5)

8.4 Discussion

We reported the course of treatment and results of endoscopic evacuation for putaminal hemorrhage in patients treated with and without AC. In this review, all cases that underwent surgical evacuation had been treated using VKAs and this represents a limitation of the analysis.

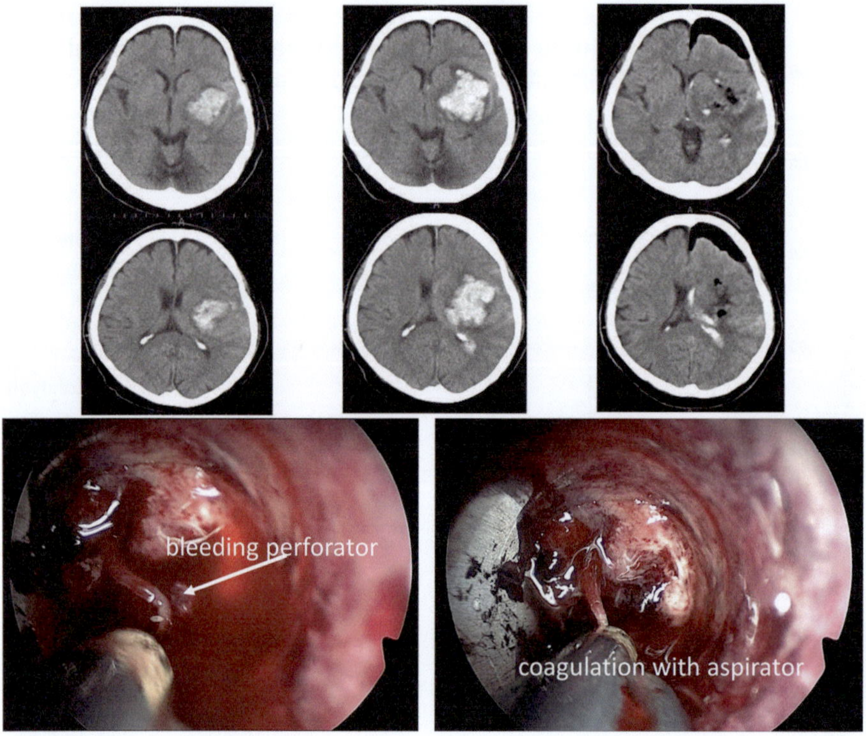

Fig. 8.2 Representative case of growing hematoma performed endoscopic evacuation with anticoagulants

In our institution, ICH related to ACs accounted for 9.7 % of cases, representing a lower frequency than the 11.9–18.4 % reported previously [2–4]. This result may be due to more prudent use of ACs in Japan. In terms of the distribution of hematoma locations, most cases involved putaminal hemorrhage located in the deep cerebrum. We performed 147 surgical evacuations (40.9 % of putaminal hemorrhages), representing a higher proportion than described in past reports. This finding may be attributable, at least in part, to the characteristics of our institution as a teaching hospital and advanced emergency medical service center.

Hemodialysis patients tend to develop large hemorrhages and most die soon after admission to hospital. In our group, five patients (71.4 % of hemodialysis patients) showed hematoma volume > 100 ml on admission. Sakamoto et al. reported that the use of an AC did not worsen outcomes for patients with ICH on hemodialysis, but the possibility of severe ICH should be considered regardless of AC use [9]. On the other hand, Wolfgang et al. reported that VKAs usage was related to hemorrhagic stroke among dialysis patients but found no association between VKA usage and ischemic stroke among dialysis patients [10]. The present review could not offer any insights into this association because of the small sample size. Randomized trials are required to assess the necessity of AC to prevent stroke in dialysis patients with NVAF.

In the present study, PT-INR on admission of 84.0 % (21/25) of ICH patients who had been receiving VKAs had been properly adjusted. In our institution, vitamin K treatment was considered for patients with AC-related ICH and PT-INR >2.0. Furthermore, cases for which surgery was indicated were treated with plasma or coagulation factor concentrate. In a previous multicenter study, Lars et al. were unable to confirm the efficacy of treatments to reverse anticoagulation effects [11]. They found a significantly lower mortality among patients treated with coagulation factors but considered that this positive effect might have been attributable to the effect of decompression by surgical evacuation. Compared with VKAs, non-VKA oral ACs (novel oral ACs; NOACs) carry a substantially lower risk of intracranial hemorrhage. A recent report found that patients with NOAC-related ICH showed smaller ICH volumes and better clinical outcomes compared with VKA-related ICH [12]. However, another report stated that NOAC-related ICH, although less frequent than VKA-related ICH, carried a higher mortality rate and was associated with more unfavorable outcomes, and hematoma expansion was more frequent [13]. Specific antidotes to reverse anticoagulation with NOACs are under clinical testing, but none are currently available for routine clinical practice. Novel drugs designed to reverse the AC effects of factor Xa inhibitors have recently been developed, and proof of efficacy in randomized trials is expected [14].

The lack of significant differences in the present study seem likely to be attributable to the small sample size, but AC-related ICH tended to be seen in older patients with larger or growing hematomas, with a longer time needed to achieve evacuation. These conditions were unfavorable for surgical evacuation. However, the present study seemed to support the notion that endoscopic evacuation of AC-related ICH did not result in inferior outcomes compared to ICH not related to use of AC. This result indicates that the reversal of AC effects led to comparable surgical conditions in the cohorts with and without AC use. The use of NOACs was not documented in our data, and clarification of this issue is therefore required in future studies.

ICH is a destructive lesion, and prevention of hematoma growth is of paramount importance in improving overall outcomes. In addition to pharmacotherapeutic hemostasis, surgical coagulation of bleeding vessels may prove useful. As surgical evacuation is invasive, even for endoscopic evacuation as a minimally invasive surgery, the preferences and consent of the patient are very important. Our surgical indications for putaminal hemorrhage currently abide by the Japanese guidelines for the management of stroke, and the target volume for hematoma is ≥31 ml, but prediction of hematoma growth may allow surgical evacuation and direct hemostasis for smaller hematomas with AC. Wada et al. reported that the spot sign on computed tomography angiography is associated with the presence and extent of hematoma progression [15]. Brouwers et al. supported the hypothesis that the spot sign offers a direct reflection of active bleeding in ICH [16, 17]. Surgical coagulation may be necessary for cases in which hematoma enlargement is expected.

8.5 Conclusion

Patients on VKAs often develop severe hemorrhage. Only 20 % of such cases are suitable for surgical evacuation. The hematoma growth rate in our study was 22 % (two of nine patients), lower than in previous reports, possibly due to speedy reversal of anticoagulation and strict control of blood pressure. Even under conditions of anticoagulation, suitable reversal may allow safe endoscopic evacuation. This means that if hematoma growth can be predicted, overall outcomes could be improved.

References

1. van Asch CJ, Luitse MJ, Rinkel GJ, van der Tweel I, Algra A, Klijn CJ. Incidence, case fatality, and functional outcome of intracerebral hemorrhage over time, according to age, sex, and ethnic origin: a systematic review and meta-analysis. Lancet Neurol. 2010;9(2):167–76.
2. Hanger HC, Fletcher VJ, Wilkinson TJ, Brown AJ, Frampton CM, Sainsbury R. Effect of aspirin and warfarin on early survival after intracerebral haemorrhage. J Neurol. 2008;255(3):347–52.
3. Stead LG, Jain A, Bellolio MF, Odufuye AO, Dhillon RK, Manivannan V, Gilmore RM, Rabinstein AA, Chandra R, Serrano LA, Yerragondu N, Palamari B, Decker WW. Effect of anticoagulant and antiplatelet therapy in patients with spontaneous intra-cerebral hemorrhage: does medication use predict worse outcome? Clin Neurol Neurosurg. 2010;112(4):275–81.
4. Stein M, Misselwitz B, Hamann GF, Kolodziej M, Reinges MH, Uhl E. In-hospital mortality after pre-treatment with antiplatelet agents or oral anticoagulants and hematoma evacuation of intracerebral hematomas. J Clin Neurosci. 2016 Apr;26:42–5.
5. Mendelow AD, Gregson BA, Fernandes HM, Murray GD, Teasdale GM, Hope DT, Karimi A, Shaw MD, DH B, STICH Investigators. Early surgery versus initial conservative treatment in patients with spontaneous supratentorial intracerebral haematomas in the International Surgical Trial in Intracerebral Haemorrhage (STICH): a randomised trial. Lancet. 2005;365(9457):387–97.
6. Mendelow AD, Gregson BA, Rowan EN, Murray GD, Gholkar A, PM M, STICH II Investigators. Early surgery versus initial conservative treatment in patients with spontaneous supratentorial lobar intracerebral haematomas (STICH II): a randomised trial. Lancet. 2013;382(9890):397–408.
7. Yokosuka K, Uno M, Hirano K, Toi H, Matsuzaki K, Matsubara S. Freehand technique for putaminal hemorrhage–technical note. Neurol Med Chir (Tokyo). 2011;51(7):543–6.
8. Nagasaka T, Tsugeno M, Ikeda H, Okamoto T, Takagawa Y, Inao S, Wakabayashi T. Balanced irrigation-suction technique with a multifunctional suction cannula and its application for intraoperative hemorrhage in endoscopic evacuation of intracerebral hematomas: technical note. Neurosurgery. 2009 Oct;65(4):E826–7 discussion E827.
9. Sakamoto N, Ishikawa E, Aoki K, Uemae Y, Komatsu Y, Matsumura A. Clinical outcomes of intracerebral hemorrhage in hemodialysis patients. World Neurosurg. 2014;81(3–4):538–42.
10. Winkelmayer WC, Liu J, Setoguchi S, Choudhry NK. Effectiveness and safety of warfarin initiation in older hemodialysis patients with incident atrial fibrillation. Clin J Am Soc Nephrol. 2011 Nov;6(11):2662–8.
11. Sjöblom L, Hårdemark HG, Lindgren A, Norrving B, Fahlén M, Samuelsson M, Stigendal L, Stockelberg D, Taghavi A, Wallrup L, Wallvik J. Management and prognostic features of intracerebral hemorrhage during anticoagulant therapy: a Swedish multicenter study. Stroke. 2001;32(11):2567–74.

12. Wilson D, Charidimou A, Shakeshaft C, Ambler G, White M, Cohen H, Yousry T, Al-Shahi Salman R, Lip GY, Brown MM, Jäger HR, DJ W, CROMIS-2 Collaborators. Volume and functional outcome of intracerebral hemorrhage according to oral anticoagulant type. Neurology. 2016;86(4):360–6.
13. Purrucker JC, Haas K, Rizos T, Khan S, Wolf M, Hennerici MG, Poli S, Kleinschnitz C, Steiner T, Heuschmann PU, Veltkamp R. Early clinical and radiological course, management, and outcome of intracerebral hemorrhage related to new oral anticoagulants. JAMA Neurol. 2016 Feb 1;73(2):169–77.
14. Siegal DM, Curnutte JT, Connolly SJ, Lu G, Conley PB, Wiens BL, Mathur VS, Castillo J, Bronson MD, Leeds JM, Mar FA, Gold A, Crowther MA. Andexanet alfa for the reversal of factor Xa inhibitor activity. N Engl J Med. 2015 Dec 17;373(25):2413–24.
15. Wada R, Aviv RI, Fox AJ, Sahlas DJ, Gladstone DJ, Tomlinson G, Symons SP. CT angiography "spot sign" predicts hematoma expansion in acute intracerebral hemorrhage. Stroke. 2007 Apr;38(4):1257–62.
16. Brouwers HB, Battey TW, Musial HH, Ciura VA, Falcone GJ, Ayres AM, Vashkevich A, Schwab K, Viswanathan A, Anderson CD, Greenberg SM, Pomerantz SR, Ortiz CJ, Goldstein JN, Gonzalez RG, Rosand J, Romero JM. Rate of contrast extravasation on computed tomographic angiography predicts hematoma expansion and mortality in primary intracerebral hemorrhage. Stroke. 2015;46(9):2498–503.
17. Brouwers HB, Raffeld MR, van Nieuwenhuizen KM, Falcone GJ, Ayres AM, McNamara KA, Schwab K, Romero JM, Velthuis BK, Viswanathan A, Greenberg SM, Ogilvy CS, van der Zwan A, Rinkel GJ, Goldstein JN, Klijn CJ, Rosand J. CT angiography spot sign in intracerebral hemorrhage predicts active bleeding during surgery. Neurology. 2014;83(10):883–9.
18. Japanese Guideline for the Management of Stroke. The joint committee on guideline for the management of stroke. Tokyo: Kyowa; 2004. p. 114–8.
19. Japanese Guideline for the Management of Stroke. The joint committee on guideline for the management of stroke. Tokyo: Kyowa; 2009. p. 152–5.

MIX
Papier aus verantwortungsvollen Quellen
Paper from responsible sources
FSC® C105338

If you have any concerns about our products,
you can contact us on
ProductSafety@springernature.com

In case Publisher is established outside the EU,
the EU authorized representative is:
Springer Nature Customer Service Center GmbH
Europaplatz 3, 69115 Heidelberg, Germany

Printed by Libri Plureos GmbH
in Hamburg, Germany